W0259595

Deconstructing Health Inequity

Timothy A. Carey · Sara J. Tai ·
Robert Griffiths

Deconstructing Health Inequity

A Perceptual Control Theory Perspective

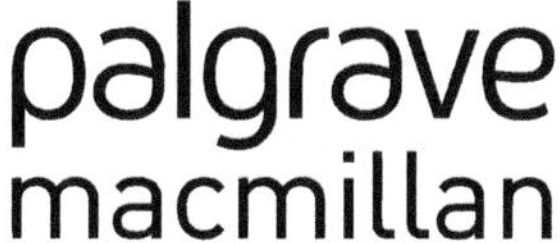

Timothy A. Carey
Institute of Global Health Equity Research
University of Global Health Equity
Kigali, Rwanda

Sara J. Tai
University of Manchester
Manchester, UK

Robert Griffiths
University of Manchester
Manchester, UK

ISBN 978-3-030-68052-7 ISBN 978-3-030-68053-4 (eBook)
https://doi.org/10.1007/978-3-030-68053-4

This Palgrave Macmillan imprint is published by the registered company Springer Nature Switzerland AG
The registered company address is: Gewerbestrasse 11, 6330 Cham, Switzerland

Foreword

In recent years concerns about increasing inequality have animated the study of social and health disparities. The considerable growth of research in this area has produced an impressive body of literature focussed on the proportional differences in adverse social and health outcomes found among geographic regions, usually wealthy countries, as well as within demographic groups, typically categorised by gender, race, ethnicity, and sexual orientation. Disparities research encompasses a wide range of problems including, mental illness, homicide, imprisonment, infant mortality, alcoholism, drug addiction, life expectancy, school dropouts, obesity, and single parenthood. Efforts to explain these problems frequently attribute the proportional differences that appear in both geographic and demographic studies to abstract structural forces. On the demographic level, for example, disparities among racial groups are often depicted as resulting from systematic barriers of institutionalised racism. And the presumed impact of economic inequality exemplifies the conventional explanation for health disparities among geographic regions. Concentrating on the latter, Timothy Carey, Sara Tai, and Robert Griffiths' book poses a formidable intellectual challenge to the prevailing assumptions that undergird the health inequities literature in particular and the disparities research in general.

Deconstructing Health Inequity: A Perceptual Control Theory Perspective is a nuanced study that illuminates the theoretical, logical, and empirical limitations, which pervade the health inequities research. On a theoretical level the analysis draws attention to the classic issue concerning the impact of structure and agency on human behaviour. From a structural perspective, individual outcomes are seen to be governed by abstract forces (e.g. class, institutionalised racism, economic inequality) emanating from the social structure; from the perspective of agency, outcomes are seen as more influenced by subjective responses to the environmental context in which one exists.

Carey, Tai, and Griffiths' analysis underscores the extent to which the abstract forces of structural theory dominate the explanation of health inequities. Seeking to clarify the theoretical basis for the prevailing explanation of health inequities, they ask the logical question: What is the causal link between economic inequality and adverse health outcomes? According to Richard Wilkinson and Kate Pickett's widely cited research, the standard answer is that income inequality generates psychological stress, which is empirically shown to have deleterious effects on physical and mental health. Really, ask Carey, Tai, and Griffiths: "Are we really that fickle as a species that we can become psychologically and socially debilitated, as well as seriously compromised by life-threatening physical health conditions, at the idea of people doing better than us?" And how does this causal line of reasoning square with Wilkinson and Pickett's finding that people tend to compare themselves with others who were similar to them, not those considerably higher on the economic ladder or the reality that most people do not know the degree of inequality in their country, how much it is changing and where they place in the income distribution. Stress may cause illness, but there is no empirical evidence that inequality (not abject poverty) causes stress.

This persuasive analysis of the implausible line of reasoning in the economic-inequality-health-inequities chain of causality is followed by the authors' painstaking examination of the empirical evidence, which reveals a body of research racked by methodological weakness, statistical anomalies, contradictory findings, and a general absence of conceptual clarity. Indeed, their findings lend detailed substantive verification to an earlier review of 98 studies that reports "little support for the idea that income inequality is a major, generalizable determinant of population health differences within or between rich countries".[1]

[1] Lynch, J., Smith, G. D., Harper, S., Hillemeier, M., Ross, N., Kaplan, G. A., et al. (2004). Is income inequality a determinant of population health: part 1. A systematic review. Milbank Quarterly, 82(1), 5–99.

Going beyond the deconstruction of health inequities, as the book's subtitle signals, the authors introduce an alternative approach to conceptualising the problem. In contrast to the dominant perspective of structural theory, they argue for examining health inequities through the alternative lens of agency as expressed in perceptual control theory. This perspective involves seeing health as essentially an individual affair and shifting the variable of individual control to centre stage of health outcomes. The extent to which perceptual control theory can deliver a precise scientific understanding of health inequities is for the reader to decide.

Deconstructing Health Inequity raises intriguing questions about the theoretical and empirical foundations of disparities research. It is a rigorous application of critical thinking that elevates the analysis of economic inequality and health inequities to a new level.

Berkeley, CA, USA Neil Gilbert

Neil Gilbert is the Milton and Gertrude Chernin Professor of Social Welfare at the University of California, Berkeley.

Preface

A no-holds-barred-warning of what's ahead.

We hadn't originally planned a Preface for this book, however, some very useful suggestions by two anonymous reviewers encouraged us to see the value in pre-empting what you might be about to encounter.

There is a Congolese saying that:

No matter how hard you throw a dead fish in the water, it still won't swim.[1]

We think this wisdom is a fitting way to set the context for the Preface. In many ways, this short introduction is a warning of what lies ahead. This book is about letting go of that fish so it can drift away.

We are not even recommending seeking another fish from the same body of water. Fundamentally, this book is a suggestion that we visit an alternative body of water where there are different fish, even fish that swim against the current. There might even be creatures we haven't yet anticipated.

If you are satisfied with the current state of play in the health inequity field, this book will not be for you. You might think that there is more

[1] Stearns, J. K. (2011). *Dancing in the glory of monsters: The collapse of the Congo and the Great War of Africa*. New York: PublicAffairs.

work to do in the sense of clarifying concepts, refining theories, identifying mechanisms, and resolving empirical anomalies. Overall though, you perhaps think that the field is generally moving in the right direction, incrementally constructing its knowledge base and addressing problems of inequity.

We don't agree.

So, as candidly as possible, we want to let you know, that if the above sentences provide a more or less accurate portrayal of your attitude and approach, you might *not* want to read any further. If you're not inclined to consider radically overhauling the foundational assumptions of the field, you are likely to be more irritated than inspired by our words. You might even form the impression that we are disingenuous peddlers of snake-oil and other potions.

More than anything, this book is a description of some of our experiences as we studied more about health inequity. As experienced health practitioners and researchers with a strong sense of social justice, we wanted to understand the important conclusions being offered.

The more we discussed and deliberated over ideas within the field of health inequity, however, the greater was our sense of bewilderment. We approached the field from the theoretical perspective identified in the subtitle of this book—Perceptual Control Theory—so we were openly bringing an established set of premises to our learning.

We think this particular theoretical lens has something to offer. Something monumental in fact. Our brash suggestion is that *inequity, per se, is* ***not*** *the problem*. We go to some lengths throughout the book to explain this position. Instead, we offer, that *disrupted control* ***is*** *the problem*. Addressing inequity *directly* will only correct disrupted control *indirectly*. Addressing control directly, however, will *necessarily* correct inequity wherever it is a problem. Health inequity, income inequity, social inequity, inequity of opportunity, and other forms of inequity could all be dealt a knockout blow if we can ever figure out how controlling creatures can inhabit the same environment without hindering, and perhaps even helping, each other's controlling efforts.

So, there you have it. That's where we are coming from.

In this book, we offer an invitation to contemplate what possibilities might emerge from considering health inequity through a lens that is radically distinct and disconnected from the current view.

Therefore, in this book, we *don't* provide an exhaustive overview of the health inequity field that demonstrates how wholeheartedly we have engaged with the current body of knowledge. We *do* provide a summary of the sources we have studied and we're reasonably sure that we haven't neglected any major contributing idea or school of thought but there will no doubt be one or more authors we haven't considered in detail.

We also *don't* offer prescriptive solutions or a detailed plan about what to do next. This book is about alternative questions we might form when wearing entirely different glasses. Our ambition is that the questions we pose and the preliminary suggestions we sketch will energise other researchers working in this field.

In the book, we *don't* allocate effort to persuading or cajoling you that these ideas are concepts you should cherish and adopt. Our priority has been to ensure that the material we present is as accurate and precise as we can make it. For the reasons we have outlined above, we are very aware that this will not be a book for all readers, so we have endeavoured to steer away from efforts to convince you. We did strive, however, to present enough information in an accessible manner so that you could convince yourself if that is what you want to do. The references we provide might assist further with that.

We have not set out to be unnecessarily provocative or heretical. That said, sometimes, considered and systematic disruption can be exactly what is needed. Perhaps for some, this book will frustrate, provoke, and unsettle. From that upheaval, new insights might sprout and flourish. If that is you, we hope to meet somewhere along the path to unknown places. Such an encounter will more than compensate for the many for whom this book offers little.

Inequity is one of the greatest scourges of our time. It is too important for complacency. Humanity's vast potential is at stake. For those with a penchant for swimming against the tide who are curious about what lies upstream, there are different waterways yet to be discovered and explored.

We have barely dipped in our toes, but the invitation remains. A more equitable, socially just world could be ours to create if we can turn away from the scene that currently dominates our view to contemplate a different territory.

Kigali, Rwanda — Timothy A. Carey
Manchester, UK — Sara J. Tai
Manchester, UK — Robert Griffiths

Contents

About the Authors

Professor Timothy A. Carey
Director Institute of Global Health Equity Research and Andrew Weiss Chair of Research in Global Health.
University of Global Health Equity, Rwanda.
Fulbright Scholar.
Author of *Patient-Perspective Care: A New Paradigm for Health Services and Systems* and *Principles-Based Counselling and Psychotherapy: A Method of Levels approach.*

Dr. Sara J. Tai
Senior Lecturer in Clinical Psychology.
University of Manchester.
Consultant Clinical Psychologist.
Greater Manchester Mental Health NHS Foundation Trust, UK.
Author of *Principles-Based Counselling and Psychotherapy: A Method of Levels approach.*

Dr. Robert Griffiths
Director Mental Health Nursing Research Unit.
Clinical Research Fellow in Mental Health Nursing.
Greater Manchester Mental Health NHS Foundation Trust, UK.
Honorary Teaching Fellow.
Division of Nursing, Midwifery and Social Work.
University of Manchester, UK.

List of Figures

List of Tables

CHAPTER 1

Beginning the Search for Answers

The true measure of any society can be found in how it treats its most vulnerable members. Mahatma Gandhi

Sometimes, some things just don't add up. For us, health inequity is one of those things.

We have a lot of expertise in the field of mental health. Collectively, we have accumulated decades of experience working in different settings with different people. We've worked in numerous inner-city services, as well as rural and underserved communities, in places such as England, Scotland, Ireland, Australia, the United States (US), and Europe. We've also worked in remote and very remote communities of the central Australian desert. Since the beginning of 2020, Tim (first author) has been working at the University of Global Health Equity in Rwanda. We've worked in primary care, secondary care, schools, inpatient wards, and prisons. We've worked with people from a range of different cultural and ethnic backgrounds, and with a wide range of psychological and social difficulties. We've developed and conducted many hours of training for other health professionals and have provided countless hours of supervision for different researchers and clinicians. We've created and evaluated innovations such as patient-led appointment scheduling, an effective and efficient first-person perspective a-diagnostic cognitive therapy, an online mental health university course, self-care training for health professionals, and smart phone apps. Almost our entire professional lives, and a good

T. A. Carey et al., *Deconstructing Health Inequity*,
https://doi.org/10.1007/978-3-030-68053-4_1

deal of our personal ones, have been geared towards helping ourselves and other people live contented lives.

Entering the Health Inequity Field

Given our interest in effective forms of helping, we recognised that it was important to not only focus on helping people individually or in small homogenous groups, but to also consider themes and patterns in the nature of peoples' problems more generally, and the implications that those patterns might have for the help that could be provided. So, addressing matters such as social justice and inequity on a broader scale became extremely relevant and interesting to us. We became well acquainted with the social determinants of health, and we were encouraged by authorities such as Smith, Bambra, and Hill (2016) who suggested that, since health inequities were linked to matters of social justice, those with expertise in psychology had a responsibility to both ask, and address, political questions related to the factors and circumstances responsible for the presence of psychosocial stressors.

Our initial learnings, however, as we entered the inequity area, puzzled us. We were interested, but not astonished, at the reported link between income inequity and population health (e.g. Babones, 2008; Smith et al., 2016). The negative relationship between these two variables has been a topic of scientific enquiry since at least the mid-1970s (Baek & Kim, 2018). We were surprised, however, by some of the claims that were made about the extent to which inequity, primarily income inequity, made people status conscious, raised stress levels, and created a multiplicity of psychological and social problems (e.g., Wilkinson & Pickett, 2010). These problems extended to serious matters including murder and violence. Apparently, the greater the income inequity of a developed nation—that is, the wider the gap between those with the most money and those with the least—the more serious we can expect individual problems of not only physical, but also social and psychological functioning, to be. According to leaders in this area, these problems affect not only the poor, but also those who are wealthy (Wilkinson & Pickett, 2018). Moreover, people from different countries in similar categories of education, social class, or income do better in those countries where the income differential gap is narrower rather than in countries where it is wider (Wilkinson & Pickett, 2010). So, a high-income earner in a more income-equal country will enjoy better physical, psychological, and social functioning than a person with a similar income in a less income-equal country (Wilkinson & Pickett, 2010).

Although the literature we initially encountered was supported by empirical evidence, it didn't fit with our clinical, research, or other professional experience. The distressed people we worked with didn't generally describe their angst in terms of the things identified as distressing in the inequity literature. Our clients, for example, seemed to be bothered by matters other than the fact that the car in their neighbour's garage cost more than theirs, or that the size of their plasma screen TV seemed puny compared to the one owned by the family who just moved in across the road.

Because our new learning didn't map easily onto our experiences, we continued to explore. We were sure there was something, or some things, we were missing or weren't understanding, and we wanted to resolve our confusion. This book is the result of that quest.

Fundamentally, we were baffled. The importance of income inequity, for example, has led some world leaders to describe it as the defining challenge of our time and the root of social problems (Gilbert, 2016; Wilkinson & Pickett, 2017). Why is inequity the problem it is portrayed to be? To state it more clearly, the two fundamental questions that guided our interrogation of the literature and most of our discussions on this topic were:

1. Why is inequity *necessarily* a problem?

and

2. Why has it been so difficult to resolve?

One thing was clear to us by now. The problem was definitely not due to a lack of resources. The problem, primarily, seemed to be one of distribution. Hickel (2017, p. 47), for example, points out that "Hunger is not a problem of lack. It is a problem of distribution. A disproportionate amount of the world's food ends up flowing to rich countries, where much of it ends up as waste." According to Hickel (2017), enough food is produced each year so that every global citizen could consume 3000 calories daily.

So, why should it matter if the person in the apartment across the hall earns more than you, or if other parents from your child's class go abroad for their holidays? Are we really that fickle as a species that we can become psychologically and socially debilitated, as well as seriously compromised by life-threatening physical health conditions, at the idea of people doing better than us? And if that's the case, why is it apparently so much worse in societies where those with the least money, and those with the most money, are a long way apart? Do people in a given society have any idea of the incomes of their poorest and richest residents?

To help us resolve our growing sense of bewilderment, we constructed a table to think through some of the information we encountered (see Table 1.1). In simplistic terms, our understanding of the general idea being communicated is that, in countries where there is a large difference between the richest and the poorest, and particularly in developed countries, there is a raft of serious physical, psychological, and social problems that affect everyone on the income continuum, from the ones at the very bottom to those at the pinnacle. In countries where the difference between the richest and the poorest is not so great, there are fewer problems. Since a lot of the research seems to draw a distinction between the developed and developing nations, for the purpose of this thought exercise, we focus on developed countries.

The conclusions we reached as we mulled over these ideas were that health and social living in Country A (see Table 1.1) would be much worse than in Countries B and C, because Country A has startling income inequity compared with the other two countries (14 compared with 3 on the fictitious scale we are using for the point of this exercise). Health and

Table 1.1 An illustration of the way in which income inequities could manifest in different developed countries

Income Inequity	Country	*Income Units		Income Inequity Measure
		Poorest	Richest	
High	A	1	15	14
Low	B	2	5	3
	C	9	12	3

*These are hypothetical income units for the purpose of illustration with lower numbers indicating less income, and higher numbers indicating greater income.

social living in Countries B and C, however, would be similar because they have the same level of income inequity even though they have very different average income levels. Moreover, the health and social functioning of people from Country A who have 12 units of income would be worse than people in Country C with the same 12 units of income, because they are situated within a country with high income inequity and, apparently, relative, rather than absolute income, is what is important. Seemingly, when groups of people with the same income are compared, people do worse in less equal societies compared to more equal societies (Wilkinson & Pickett, 2010). Similarly, the health and social functioning of someone in Country B with 3 units of income would be better than the health and social functioning of someone in Country A with 3 units of income (see Table 1.1).

This reasoning didn't make sense to us. We continued to entertain the idea that we were misunderstanding the literature and unintentionally building straw men which we could subsequently knock down. The more we read, however, the more our initial assumptions seemed to be confirmed.

Before going any further, we should comment on the terms *inequity* and *inequality*. Efforts have been made in some places to draw a distinction between the terms. Arcaya, Arcaya, and Subramanian (2015, p. 2), for example, explain:

> *The key distinction between the terms inequality and inequity is that the former is simply a dimensional description employed whenever quantities are unequal, while the latter requires passing a moral judgment that the inequality is wrong.*

Some of the most high-profile writers in this area, however, appear to frame problems in terms of inequality, rather than inequity (Marmot, 2015; Wilkinson & Pickett, 2010). Smith et al. (2016) suggest that, in different contexts, different terms are used to refer to the same thing. Specifically, they offer that in the US and Canada the term "health disparities" is used while in low- and middle-income countries (LMICs) the term "health inequities" is preferred (Smith et al., 2016). For the purposes of this book, we use "health inequity" because that seemed to us to be the most commonly used term in the literature.

A Bias Towards Understanding How People Work

One other thing you should know about us at the beginning of this book is that we all share an abiding interest in understanding how people work. We use the term "work" here in the sense of how our bodies do what they do to continually create the lives we live, not in the occupational sense of building a career or earning enough money to make ends meet. Appreciating the mechanics and necessary processes that allow people to navigate their days, the factors that enable them to thrive, and all the things that can compromise that flourishing are some of the favourite things we like to discuss, research, teach, and write about, as well as apply in our clinical practice. We will provide a lot more detail about these ideas in Chapter 3. And, in fact, the majority of this book is the culmination of where our myriad queries, conversations, and cogitations took us, as we discovered, then pondered, the various inequity ideas in the context of our primary preference for understanding how humans work.

A Lack of Agreement in the Field

To find a way out of the conceptual labyrinth in which we had become ensnared, we read widely, and discussed and debated the various findings we encountered. Before too long, we were struck by the general lack of consensus in the field. While almost everyone agrees that inequity is counterproductive—although even here some people think a certain amount of inequity is inevitable with the important issues being how it comes about and how much is acceptable (Gilbert, 2016; Marmot, 2015; OECD, 2008)—beyond this general level of agreement, there are rampant differences of opinion.

Could Perspective Be Part of the Problem?

As our learning continued, it became more and more apparent, that the current prevailing perspective might be as much of a problem as any particular method or research finding in the inequity realm. It seemed like something similar to the story of the "blind men and the elephant" might be occurring. We were also reminded of the difficulties confronted by the geocentric astronomers of centuries past as they tried to improve the accuracy of their models of celestial bodies circling the earth. The relevance here was that problems that arose were not due to limitations in the capabilities of the astronomers or the equipment at their disposal. The problem was perspective. It was the astronomers' frame of reference that needed altering, not the methods they used, or the way they used them. Once a heliocentric model of the solar system became accepted, the problems inherent in the geocentric perspective became redundant, and different questions required answering.

We wondered if something similar was occurring in the inequity field.

As we continued to search for answers, we applied our understanding of human functioning to all that we encountered. In this book, therefore, we don't aim to provide answers as much as we'd like to table a possible constructive direction in which innovative, original questions could be formulated to yield novel answers. We're wondering, if it would make a difference to the way in which inequity is understood, investigated, and addressed, if human nature was considered *this* way, rather than from the current prevailing perspective. The information in this book is a detailed explanation and analysis of *this* applied to inequity.

We openly acknowledge our newness to the health inequity field and our lack of recognised authority in this area. A fresh and unfamiliar approach, however, could be considered an advantage. With backgrounds in psychological knowledge and research, and an understanding of the way in which individuals function as purposive agents embedded in social environments, we have been able to consider the work in this area in ways that might, ultimately, be considered unconventionally constructive. It is this unfamiliar point of view that we're suggesting could offer an alternative and useful approach to people who are looking for different options in addressing problems of inequity.

Sharing Our Journey

For the remainder of this chapter we'll highlight, generally, the main ideas we've discovered in the health inequity domain. In the next chapter, we'll provide a little more detail of some of the places in which there seems to be a generous dollop of disharmony. These two early chapters are provided to set a context, and to indicate where some of the main divisions exist. Our purpose in writing this book was not to chronicle in a fine-grained way all that has been done and is known in the inequity terrain. Rather, we'd like to provide enough information for you to judge for yourself the soundness (or otherwise) of our reasoning. We also wanted to justify why we thought a renovation of the area was warranted, so that we could then describe some of the possibilities for where a new approach might lead.

In Chapter 3 we introduce our understanding of how people function. Chapter 4 explores the implications of this understanding for the way in which we define health. In Chapters 5 and 6 we spend time looking closely at the research strategies and tactics that define the inequity domain in terms of concepts such as causality and statistical significance and we provide some alternative ideas. Chapter 7 takes a case study approach with one important paper to demonstrate that many of the field's findings are not wrong as much as they are incomplete. In Chapter 8 we turn our gaze from research to practice and outline some of the ways our ideas might inform current approaches to healthcare and the associated practices.

To conclude the book in a way that we could be satisfied with, we wanted to do as much as we could to answer the important "so what?" question. So, in Chapter 9, the final chapter, we stretch our wonderings a little further. We don't think we ever stray into the ludicrous or the implausible but that might not be our judgement to make.

So, now that you have a sense of what lies ahead, let's get down to business …

Before we can sensibly discuss where an alternative present time could be and what it might look like, however, it is important to appreciate the state of our current present time with regard to health inequity. It is to the task of providing our general impression of the existing state of knowledge to which we now turn.

The Link Between Income Inequity and Health Outcomes

While the characteristics of a contented life, and what promotes and impedes it, have interested us for the longest time, we think of our reading about the link between income inequity and a plethora of psychological and social problems as the place where this particular part of our journey began. It was some of this work that perplexed us, and created the quandary we found ourselves in, so this is perhaps the most appropriate place to commence an overview of the field.

The Main Point and Some Nuances of Which to Be Aware

The general idea being conveyed by proponents of the position that income inequity and physical, psychological, and social functioning are tightly linked, is that the way we relate to each other on a societal level is strongly influenced by the scale of the income differences of that society (Wilkinson & Pickett, 2010). Apparently, within any particular country, people's health and happiness are related to their income such that wealthy people, on average, are healthier and happier than poor people (Wilkinson & Pickett, 2010).

There are at least four qualifiers which are essential to be aware of in order to appreciate the scope of this research. First, these findings apply only to more affluent countries. It appears that economic development is important for well-being in poorer countries but, as countries join the ranks of the well-to-do, economic development becomes less and less relevant to well-being (Smith et al., 2016; Wilkinson & Pickett, 2010, 2018). Bartley (2017), however, introduces an important nuance here related to the health of an individual and the health of society. Beyond a certain average income, increases in this income do not seem to improve the health of that society. The health of an individual *within a country*, however, does seem to be better if they enjoy more prestige and favourable employment conditions (Bartley, 2017).

Second, some researchers contend that it is the magnitude of income inequity which is important, *not* a wealthy country's average income (Wilkinson & Pickett, 2010). Apparently, the same effect is found in affluent countries with greater or lesser average income, such that physical, psychological, and social functioning are only weakly related to a rich country's average income (Wilkinson & Pickett, 2010). Even here, however, there are important caveats since Curran and Mahutga's (2018) work indicates that income inequity impacts most detrimentally on the population health of the *least* developed countries with no significantly harmful impact in high-income countries.

Third, the link between income inequity and different aspects of daily functioning is most strongly found when comparisons occur on larger scales such as countries, states, or regions (Pickett & Wilkinson, 2010). The link is not as obvious or robust when small local areas and communities are considered. Pickett and Wilkinson (2015) report that variations in geographical scale between different studies are a methodological consideration that influences the outcomes of those studies. When larger jurisdictions are investigated, income inequity can be considered to be an indicator of the extent of social stratification, or hierarchicalisation, that exists and, in this context, the link between income inequity and health is generally supported (Pickett & Wilkinson, 2010).

Fourth, even when the link between income inequity and physical, psychological, and social functioning can be identified, on average, in wealthier countries, for larger groupings of people, it only applies to aspects of functioning that have strong social class gradients (Wilkinson & Pickett, 2010). Apparently, cardiovascular disease and crime are included, but breast and prostate cancer are not (Wilkinson & Pickett, 2017). If you are wondering, at this point, why some problems in functioning might exhibit what are called social gradients, while others do not, you will have taken a little step into the world we experienced as mystifying as we plunged into this work.

A Closer Look at the Findings

Having established some of the parameters to the scope of this research, we can consider in more detail key findings from the literature. Wilkinson and Pickett (2010) are among a number of researchers who convey a strong interest in the social impact of income inequity. Table 1.2 provides examples from the literature of different researchers and the ways in which they report income inequity impacting on physical, psychological, and social functioning. When they measure income inequity, for example, they assert that they are actually measuring indicators of the degree to which a society is hierarchicalised such as social distance and social stratification. The hierarchy is important because disparities in those aspects of functioning that are affected by a social gradient impact not only on the poor, but also on the wealthy. Those who are only reasonably well-off, for example, have shorter lives than those who are extremely wealthy (Wilkinson & Pickett, 2010). The gradient effect only emerges, however, when group, rather than individual, data are considered. Without that qualifier, one could reasonably expect from Wilkinson and Pickett's (2010) findings that the oldest person in any given (affluent) society would be the wealthiest and, similarly, that the person at the top of the money pile would live to be the oldest member of that society. With that detail clarified, the conclusion that inequity has effects throughout society, not just for poor people, is emphasised in a number of sources (Wilkinson & Pickett, 2010, 2018).

Table 1.2 Examples from the literature of aspects of physical, psychological, and social functioning that are reported to be linked to income inequity

Source	Different Features of Functioning
Babones, 2008	Life expectancy; infant mortality; murder rates; population health
Baek & Kim, 2018	Infant mortality
Bartley, 2017	Unemployment benefits; public health services; education; housing; transport; life expectancy; social pathology; competition and cooperation; trust; criminal behavior; pollution; traffic hazards
Bezruchka, 2014	Mortality levels; infant death rates
Curran & Mahutga, 2018	Population health
Frank, 2014	Bankruptcy rates; divorce rates; commute times
Kragten & Rozer, 2017	Life expectancy; self-rated health; social trust
Marmot, 2015	Social cohesion; economic growth
OECD, 2008	Social mobility; political influence of the wealthy; economic performance; capacity to act collectively; health outcomes; educational outcomes
OECD, 2011	Social mobility; opportunity; political stability; economic performance
Patel et al., 2018	Mental health
Pickett & Wilkinson, 2010	Mental illness; physical health; trust; violence
Pickett & Wilkinson, 2015	Life expectancy; mental illness; obesity; infant mortality; teenage births; homicides; imprisonment; educational attainment; distrust; social mobility
Schneider, 2019	Life satisfaction; subjective social status; wellbeing
Smith et al., 2016	Health; mortality; environmental issues
Stiglitz, 2012	Educational opportunity; nutrition; exposure to environmental pollutants
Wilkinson, 2014	Death rates; health; obesity; infant death rates
Wilkinson & Pickett, 2010	Child wellbeing; women's obesity (the link is not as strong for men's obesity); health; status competition and status anxiety; trust; mental illness in adult women (but not adult men); use of illegal drugs such as cocaine, marijuana, and heroin; death from heart disease; deaths from homicide; illness; status insecurity; violence; divorce rates; children's aspirations (higher in unequal countries)
Wilkinson & Pickett, 2017	Life expectancy; mortality rates; life chances and trajectories of childhood; mental health
Wilkinson & Pickett, 2018	Life expectancy; infant mortality; mental illness; illicit drug use (including heroin, cocaine, amphetamines); obesity; violence (measured by homicide rates – adult and juvenile); imprisonment; trust; community life; child wellbeing; educational attainment; teenage births; social mobility; status anxiety; worries about being judged; depression; psychotic symptoms; schizophrenia; narcissistic traits; alcohol consumption; self-esteem; confidence; educational standards; participation in the arts; proportion of the labour force employed in guard labour (security staff, police, prison officers); lower productivity

Explaining Why Income Inequity Might Have the Effect That It Does

While we were intrigued about the extent of the reported association between income inequity and physical, psychological, and social functioning, we were especially surprised at the explanations given for this relationship. Wilkinson and Pickett (2018, p. xxi), for example, argue that "if well-educated people with good jobs and incomes lived with the same jobs and incomes in a more equal society, they would be likely to live a little longer and less likely to become victims of violence; their children might do a little better at school and would be less likely to become teenage parents or to develop serious drug problems". This is an example of the reasoning we were depicting in Table 1.1. Wilkinson and Pickett (2018, p. xxi) go on to suggest that the issue is "the way larger income differences across a society immerse everyone more deeply in issues of status competition and hierarchy". They explain that "these problems are driven by the stress of social status differences themselves, stresses which get worse the lower you are on the social ladder and the bigger the status differences. In effect, bigger income differences make status differences more potent" (Wilkinson & Pickett, 2018, p. xxii). In the same source, Wilkinson and Pickett (2018, p. 25) clarify their position by suggesting that although "low incomes limit what poorer people can buy, they leave status aspirations undiminished – or even heightened – by the desire to escape the stigma of low social status". They also link extreme shyness, which they acknowledge can be diagnosed as social phobia or social anxiety disorder, to income inequity, and they report that the prevalence of people diagnosed with social anxiety disorder in the US has increased over three decades from 2% to 12% of the population (Wilkinson & Pickett, 2018).

It was perhaps our familiarity with the mental health field that indicated to us that there might be something amiss with the explanatory conclusions being drawn in the inequity arena. There is, in fact, a voluminous literature outlining the many different problems with the Western biomedical approach to understanding psychological and social functioning as it is described in the fifth edition of the *Diagnostic and Statistical Manual of Mental Disorders* (DSM 5; American Psychiatric Association, APA, 2013). Timimi (2014) provides an excellent overview of some of the major problems. Social phobia was created and first introduced into the DSM system in its third edition in 1980 (Whitaker & Cosgrove, 2015). There is compelling evidence that the explosion in the identification and diagnosis of this manufactured disorder has far less to do with income inequity than with the monstrously enthusiastic (some would say aggressive) and sustained promotion of the disorder, and marketing of pharmaceutical treatments by the APA and the pharmaceutical industry (Whitaker & Cosgrove, 2015).

There are other reasons one might question the extent to which everyone in a society characterised by large income differences is stressfully consumed by status competition leading to increases in social phobia or social anxiety disorder diagnoses. Perhaps the preferences and patterns of media use by populations have something to offer here. The television show *Lifestyles of the Rich and Famous*, for example, screened from 1984 to 1995. It has been described as ushering in a new era of television programmes that brought the wealthiest people into our living rooms and paraded their lifestyles and living quarters before us. *Lifestyles* had spin-off programmes, a board game, and a video slot machine generated from its success. Would large numbers of people tune into *Lifestyles,* and the later shows it spawned, if they were all wracked with anxiety by the very same status differences each episode of these programmes ostentatiously flaunted? It is difficult to reconcile this suggested population-level self-torture with our understanding of Western life in the 1980s and 1990s. Also, some popstars have enormous followings on social media such as Twitter and Instagram. Shakira and Britney Spears, for example, have more than 50 million Twitter followers, while Justin Timberlake has more than 60 million followers. Kim Kardashian has, reportedly, 157 million followers on Instagram. We are certainly not oblivious to the problems social media can have for people's psychological and social functioning. We are tabling, however, the possibility that gaping financial and status differences might not be the widespread scourges they are sometimes reported to be, and that, in fact, some people might be buoyed rather than bothered by the trappings of the ultra-rich.

Gilbert (2016, p. 68) is also sceptical of the way in which the link between psychological stress and income inequity is explained by Wilkinson and Pickett (2010, p. 43) and refers to their suggestion as "flimsy speculation". To compound our confusion, the supposed association between psychological functioning and income inequity conflicted with other reports in the literature including Wilkinson and Pickett's later research. For example, Wilkinson and Pickett (2018) maintained that a consistent finding in their research was a strong tendency for people to compare themselves with others who were similar to them, such as work colleagues, not with people who were far away on the social ladder. To the extent that people engage in social comparisons at all, if they only compare themselves to those with whom they are similar, we could not understand the significance of a wide income gap. Perhaps part of the problem here is the application of findings obtained from population level data to individual lives.

Alternative Views About the Research

Despite the volume of research indicating a strong link between income inequity and a range of problems with physical, psychological, and social functioning, the robustness of this connection continues to be questioned. Schneider (2019), for example, describes the research findings regarding the link between income inequity and well-being as inconsistent, and indicates that the consequences of income inequity might not be as straightforward as is often reported. Smith et al. (2016) also report that the empirical basis for psychosocial explanations of the link between inequity and health have been challenged. Rozer, Kraaycamp, and Huijts (2016) empirically tested the hypothesised link between income inequity and health and found no significant relationship between national income inequity and self-rated health.

Bartley (2017) describes the amount of disagreement regarding the relationship between income inequity and health as “considerable”. Furthermore, even when there is agreement regarding the relationship between income inequity and health, there is frequently concurrent *disagreement* about why this might be so (Bartley, 2017). Marmot (2015) also contends that the evidence indicating that income inequities are bad for health is weaker now than it once was. Perhaps the disagreement exists because, whatever relationship there is between income inequity and health, it is not particularly strong. Babones (2008) refers to Beckfield’s (2004) earlier work that produced from a comprehensive study, a correlation between population health and income inequity of −0.31. Although this correlation was reported as highly statistically significant, a coefficient of this size does not indicate a strong relationship. It is often helpful to visualise what different correlations look like. In Fig. 1.1, we have created a scatterplot of a correlation of −0.31 between two variables, “x” and “y”. In this instance “x” could be a measure of income inequity such as the Gini coefficient (a widely used measure of inequity

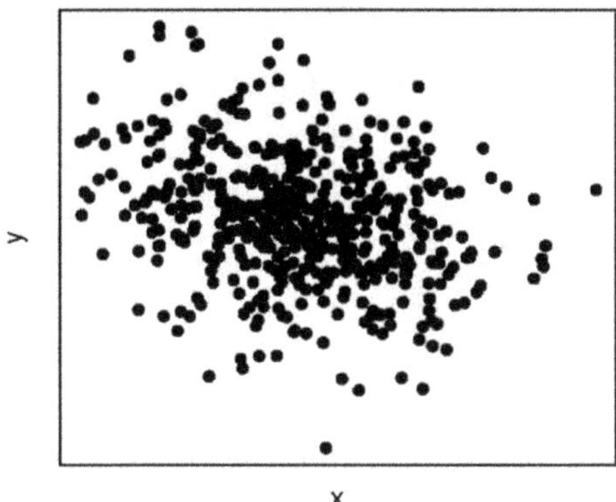

Fig. 1.1 A correlation of −0.31 between two variables *x* and *y*

whereby 0 is perfect equity, everyone has the same amount of money; and 1 is perfect inequity, one person has all the money; Starmans, Sheskin, & Bloom, 2017), and "y" could be a measure of population health such as "life expectancy". The actual scatterplot can be seen in Beckfield (2004) on page 237. Beckfield's (2004) figure is not dissimilar to the scatterplot in Fig. 1.1.

The most striking characteristic of a scatterplot for a correlation of the magnitude Beckfield (2004) reports is just exactly how much scatter there is. There is a lot more scatter than plot. The amount of scatter is important because that determines how much information you might be able to discern from one variable, by knowing a value of the other variable. In this instance, if we were to *plot* an arbitrary value of "x" (which we might think of as income inequity represented by the Gini coefficient) and draw a vertical line from that value, you might be able to appreciate just how much *scatter* there is for the "y" values (which in this example is health represented by life expectancy) along this line. Figure 1.2 illustrates this point with a red vertical line for some arbitrarily chosen value of the Gini coefficient. All the different points along that line represent the range of different values of individual life expectancy (or health) *for the same value* of income inequity (see Fig. 1.2). So, knowing the value of a particular Gini coefficient doesn't really tell you very much about what to expect regarding population health or life expectancy.

Even with topics of the nature of the relationship aside, ten years after Babones (2008), Blazquez-Fernandez, Cantarero-Prieto, and Pascual-Saez (2018) reported that, in their study, income inequity in developed

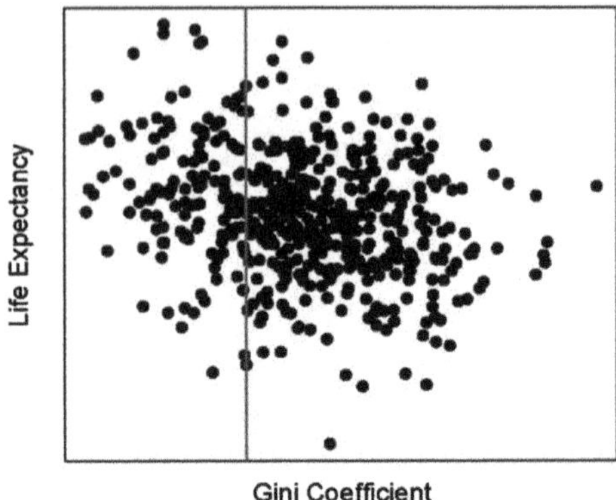

Fig. 1.2 Examining different values of health (life expectancy) for a particular value of income inequity (Gini coefficient)

countries did not significantly reduce health. Blazquez-Fernandez et al. (2018) describe an extraordinary lack of scientific consensus on the relationship between income inequity and health. Baek and Kim (2018) report that the proposal that income inequity, rather than economic growth, determines population health in wealthy countries is a hypothesis that has been widely debated over a long period of time. In their study, the statistical significance of the relationship between life expectancy and income inequity disappeared when control variables such as education and public health spending were added.

In particular, with regard to the psychosocial explanation of health differences between more and less equal countries, Bartley (2017) regards the emphasis on people's perception of their relative status in a social hierarchy as "controversial". To reinforce the query we introduced earlier, Bartley (2017) questions whether people's concern regarding the impressiveness of their car, relative to their neighbour's, is so great that it compromises their health. To be clear, Bartley (2017) is not suggesting that a relationship between income inequity and health does not exist, but she does question whether explanations of relative deprivation and aroused emotions are necessary to explain it. Stiglitz (2012) also doesn't look for explanations of inequity beyond government policies in terms of what governments do, as well as what they fail to do. Similarly, Hickel (2017) provides evidence of the power of government policies in driving social inequity to unprecedented levels in both the US and the United Kingdom (UK). Resolution of some of the current dissonance, to the extent that it is possible, has important practical implications. With regard to policy, for example, Blazquez-Fernandez et al. (2018) report that the results of their study indicate that directing policies and resources towards income inequity is *not* likely to benefit population health in affluent societies. Given the amount of resources allocated to addressing problems perceived to be caused by inequity, driven by policies such as the United Nation's (UN) Sustainable Development Goals (UN, 2015), Blazques-Fernandez et al.'s (2018) point is somewhat alarming.

Pausing to Reflect

At this stage of our exploration and learning we were impressed to the point of being overwhelmed by the extent of the dissent existing in this important area. Is inequity of any sort, detrimental to human functioning? We felt intuitively that it was, but were not able to say why beyond a moral sense of fairness and justice. Why should someone's heart or pancreas be concerned about where the body in which they are ensconced is positioned in a social hierarchy? There seemed to be little agreement in the literature about what exactly the problem was, and even more importantly, why it was a problem. We continued, therefore, to search for greater clarity. Chapter 2 provides details of that search.

References

American Psychiatric Association. (2013). *Diagnostic and statistical manual of mental disorders* (5th ed.). Washington, DC: American Psychiatric Association.

Arcaya, M. C., Arcaya, A. L., & Subramanian, S. V. (2015). Inequalities in health: Definitions, concepts, and theories. *Global Health Action, 38*(4), 261–271. https://doi.org/10.3402/gha.v8.27106.

Babones, S. J. (2008). Income inequality and population health: Correlation and causality. *Social Science and Medicine, 66*, 1614–1626.

Baek, S.-H., & Kim, K.-T. (2018). Retesting the income inequality hypothesis: Pooled time-series-cross-section regression with a new statistical case selection method. *Asian Social Work and Policy Review, 12*, 191–199. https://doi.org/10.1111/aswp.12150.

Bartley, M. (2017). *Health inequality: An introduction to concepts, theories and methods* (2nd ed.). Cambridge: Polity Press.

Beckfield, J. (2004). Does income inequality harm health? Now cross-national evidence. *Journal of Health and Social Behavior, 45*(3), 231–248.

Bezruchka, S. (2014). Inequality kills. In D. C. Johnston (Ed.), *Divided: The perils of our growing inequality* (pp. 190–198). New York: The New Press.

Blazquez-Fernandez, C., Cantarero-Prieto, D., & Pascual-Saez, M. (2018). Does rising income inequality reduce life expectancy? New evidence for 26 European countries (1995–2014). *Global Economic Review: Perspectives on East Asian Economies and Industries, 47*(4), 464–479. https://doi.org/10.1080/1226508X.2018.1526098.

Curran, M., & Mahutga, M. C. (2018). Income inequality and population health: A global gradient? *Journal of Health and Social Behavior, 59*(4), 536–553.

Frank, R. H. (2014). How gains at the top injure the middle class. In D. C. Johnston (Ed.), *Divided: The perils of our growing inequality* (pp. 35–42). New York: The New Press.

Gilbert, N. (2016). *Never enough: Capitalism and the progressive spirit*. Oxford: Oxford University Press.

Hickel, J. (2017). *The divide: A brief guide to global inequality and its solutions*. London: Penguin Random House.

Kragten, N., & Rozer, J. (2017). The income inequality hypothesis revisited: Assessing the hypothesis using four methodological approaches. *Social Indicators Research, 131,* 1015–1033.

Marmot, M. (2015). *The health gap: The challenge of an unequal world*. London: Bloomsbury.

OECD. (2008). *Growing unequal? Income distribution and poverty in OECD countries*. Paris: OECD Publishing.

OECD. (2011). *Divided we stand: Why inequality keeps rising*. Paris: OECD Publishing. http://dxdoi.org/10.1787/97264119536-en.

Patel, V., Burns, J. K., Dhingra, M., Tarver, L., Kohrt, B. A., & Lund, C. (2018). Income inequality and depression: A systematic review and meta-analysis of the association and a scoping review of mechanisms. *World Psychiatry, 17*(1), 76–89.

Pickett, K. E., & Wilkinson, R. G. (2010). Inequality: An underacknowledged source of mental illness and distress. *The British Journal of Psychiatry, 197,* 426–428. https://doi.org/10.1192/bjp.bp.109.072066.

Pickett, K. E., & Wilkinson, R. G. (2015). Income inequality and health: A causal review. *Social Science and Medicine, 128,* 316–326.

Rozer, J., Kraaykamp, G., & Huijts, T. (2016). National income inequality and self-rated health: The differing impact of individual social trust across 89 countries. *European Societies, 18*(3), 245–263. https://doi.org/10.1080/14616696.2016.1153697.

Schneider, S. M. (2019). Why income inequality is dissatisfying—Perceptions of social status and the inequality-satisfaction link in Europe. *European Sociological Review, 35*(3), 409–430. https://doi.org/10.1093/esr/jcz003.

Smith, K. E., Bambra, C., & Hill, S. (2016). Background and introduction: UK experiences of health inequalities. In K. E. Smith, S. Hill, & C. Bambra (Eds.), *Health inequalities: Critical perspectives* (pp. 1–21). Oxford: Oxford University Press.

Starmans, C., Sheskin, M., & Bloom, P. (2017). Why people prefer unequal societies. *Nature Human Behavior, 1*(0082). https://doi.org/10.1038/s41562-017-0082.

Stiglitz, J. E. (2012). *The price of inequality*. London: Penguin.

Timimi, S. (2014). No more psychiatric labels: Why formal psychiatric diagnostic systems should be abolished. *International Journal of Clinical and Health Psychology, 14,* 208–215.

UN. (2015). *United Nations Transforming Our World: The 2030 Agenda for Sustainable Development. A/RES/70/1*. United Nations (Vol. 16301). Accessed 30 September 2020. https://www.un.org/en/development/desa/population/migration/generalassembly/docs/globalcompact/A_RES_70_1_E.pdf.

Whitaker, R., & Cosgrove, L. (2015). *Psychiatry under the influence: Institutional corruption, social injury, and prescription for reform*. New York: Palgrave Macmillan.

Wilkinson, R. G. (2014). Health and income inequalities are linked. In D. C. Johnston (Ed.), *Divided: The perils of our growing inequality* (pp. 161–163). New York: The New Press.

Wilkinson, R. G., & Pickett, K. E. (2010). *The spirit level: Why equality is better for everyone*. London: Penguin Books.

Wilkinson, R. G., & Pickett, K. E. (2017). The enemy between us: The psychological and social costs of inequality. *European Journal of Social Psychology, 47,* 11–24.

Wilkinson, R. G., & Pickett, K. E. (2018). *The Inner level: How more equal societies reduce stress, restore sanity and improve everyone's well-being*. London: Penguin Random House.

CHAPTER 2

A Closer Look at the Scientific Literature

Scientists have learned to respect nothing but evidence, and to believe that their highest duty lies in submitting to it however it may jar against their inclinations. Thomas Huxley

Things added up less to us now than they had when we first began to interrogate the health inequity literature, with the questions we articulated at the end of Chapter 1 demanding our attention.

To assist in compiling the information in this chapter, and to communicate it as clearly and coherently as possible, we have divided the information into several sections. It will be apparent, as you read, that there is overlap between the sections. We felt, however, there were core ideas in each section that were important to highlight and emphasise.

The Contribution of Theoretical Frameworks

One could argue that the development and refinement of theoretical frameworks is an important component of all serious scientific pursuits. The unique contribution of science is "its respect for the power of empirical evidence to shape and change our theories, and reliance on the practices of critical scrutiny by our peers to catch our mistakes if we do not" (McIntyre, 2019, p. 317). A willingness to change theories on the basis of evidence is an exclusive and distinguishing hallmark of science (McIntyre, 2019).

T. A. Carey et al., *Deconstructing Health Inequity*,
https://doi.org/10.1007/978-3-030-68053-4_2

We have explained that we were aware of bringing our own theoretical biases to the learning we pursued. We were particularly interested, therefore, in establishing the amount of convergence there might be between the established theoretical positions in the inequity literature and our own theoretical stance. Yet, our initial explorations soon revealed a high degree of uncertainty and indecision in the theoretical explanations of health inequity.

Rozer, Kraaykamp, and Huijts (2016) suggest there is a need for clear theorising with regard to inequity to ensure that appropriate attention is paid to the range of harmful consequences that can occur for people living in an unequal society. While we unreservedly agree with Rozer et al.'s (2016) assertion of the need for clear theorising, it seemed to us that, even in this statement, there was an *a priori* assumption that inequity *is* harmful. We were eager to explore the empirical support for this assumption.

Elsewhere we have identified the importance of "meta-methods" (Carey, Huddy, & Griffiths, 2019). Meta-methods are assumptions or methods that have a strong influence on the attitudes and conduct of researchers. The "meta" nature of these influencing ideas, however, means that researchers might not always be fully aware of exactly what meta-methods they subscribe to, or the effect these beliefs have on their work. Meta-methods aside, the inconsistencies we encountered in the literature raised for us, important questions about what the fundamental components of inequity might be. Schneider (2019), for example, considers social comparison to be a key mechanism through which income inequity contributes to lower status perception.

Our reading revealed to us that the link between income inequity and health inequity was regarded by many as a hypothesis—the "income inequity hypothesis" (also known as the "Wilkinson hypothesis")—and was considered to be one of the psychosocial theories of inequity (Smith, Bambra, & Hill, 2016). Materialist theories, on the other hand, concentrate on environmental factors such as housing, and criticise psychosocial theories for shifting attention towards individuals and away from important policy considerations (Smith et al., 2016). Bartley (2017) explains that materialist theories focus on the impact social and economic conditions have on people's bodies. Theories described as neomaterialist are concerned with why, in more equal societies, people experience better health across a range of situations (Bartley, 2017). The psychosocial and neomaterialist distinctions are commonly referred to in the literature (e.g. Rozer et al., 2016) with other explanations also being noted, such as what Rozer et al. (2016) refer to as compositional mechanisms or compositional arguments, which consider the role of individual income and poverty.

Bartley (2017), however, categorises the current theories somewhat differently, arguing that the work of Wilkinson, Pickett, and others pays less attention to the individual and social groups and much more attention to the macro-social or political economy explanations. That is, these people primarily study the health of countries with different levels of welfare provisions. Other work suggests that economic development moderates the relationship between income inequity and health (Curran & Mahutga, 2018). As mentioned in Chapter 1, Curran and Mahutga (2018) found that income inequity had more harmful effects in poorer rather than richer countries.

Neomaterialists also dispute psychosocial explanations and, instead, explain the greater health enjoyed by people in more equal societies in terms of policies influencing the provision of public services (Bartley, 2017). Bartley (2017), however, is cognisant of the fact that matters such as social class, education, and income do not fully explain health status, and recommends that explanations should also account for individuals' lived environments. Somewhat consistently perhaps, Collins, McCrory, Mackenzie, and McCartney (2015) adopt a stance of not rejecting the income inequity hypothesis but going beyond it. Curran and Mahutga (2018) discuss the alternative explanations according to integrationist and neomaterialist categories. Curran and Mahutga's (2018) work emphasises the importance of neomaterialist processes, suggesting that changes to national political and institutional contexts could improve health even if income inequity remains constant.

Freeman Anderson, Bjorklund, and Rambotti (2019) hypothesise that there might be three theoretical pathways linking income inequity and individual health. They also acknowledge that the two main theoretical positions in the literature for the association between income inequity and health outcomes are relative and absolute deprivation. They clarify, however, that these positions are not mutually exclusive and can even function in conjunction with each other (Freeman Anderson et al., 2019).

Stiglitz (2012) provides an interesting and useful perspective with the "marginal productivity theory". According to Stiglitz (2012), the vast majority of the population are not jealous or envious of very rich people who have well-deserved incomes. The position of Stiglitz (2012) is that it is the way in which some fortunes are amassed that is perceived as unfair rather than the fortunes themselves. Starmans, Sheskin, and Bloom (2017), as will be explained below, also contend that it is fairness, rather than equity, that is of concern to most people.

Current theories, therefore, seem to emphasise either the individual or the environment. What appears to be missing is a coherent account of the way in which individuals influence, *and are simultaneously influenced by*, the environments they inhabit. In this regard, Elliott, Popay, and Williams (2016) recommend that the literature on the concept of control might offer useful theoretical contributions by addressing not only the functioning of the individual but also the individual situated within a community and culture.

Given the emphasis introduced earlier of sound theories for successful scientific activity (McIntyre, 2019), the ragged nature of the assortment of theories in this domain could be one of the primary reasons for the lack of substantial progress. In a consideration of social science research generally, McIntyre (2019, p. 201) insists, that "It should be recognized as the embarrassment it is that there is so much opinion, intuition, theory, and ideology". Opinion, intuition, theory, and ideology would be apt descriptors of the health inequity literature as we encountered it.

Methodological Considerations

The more we read, the more we discovered that we were by no means the first people to highlight discrepancies in the literature. Other researchers and commentators have drawn attention to the panoply of methodologies that are used in this field and point to this methodological heterogeneity as one of the contributing factors for the multitudinous inconsistencies that exist. McIntyre (2019, p. 297) underscores this point:

> *Too much social research is embarrassingly unrigorous. Not only are the methods sometimes poor, much more damning is the nonempirical attitude that lies behind them. Many allegedly scientific studies on immigration, guns, the death penalty, and other important social topics are infected by their investigator's political or ideological views, so that it is all but expected that some researchers will discover results that are squarely in line with liberal political beliefs, while others will produce conservative results that are directly opposed to them.*

The lack of consistent research findings concerning the connection between income inequity and health, and the consequent controversy in the literature regarding the nature of the relationship between income inequity and health problems, has been attributed to methodological differences (Blazquez-Fernandez, Cantarero-Prieto, & Pascual-Saez, 2018; Schneider, 2019). Freeman Anderson et al. (2019) comment on the inconclusive nature of the research that examines the link between income inequity and health, and maintain that income inequity is more nuanced than is generally proposed. The complexity regarding the way in which income inequity is defined and constructed is widely acknowledged (e.g. OECD, 2008).

At this point we would once again refer to the meta-methods (Carey et al., 2019) that, from our perspective, influence the way in which decisions are made. For example, in a study investigating the relationship between control in the home and coronary heart disease (CHD), Chandola, Kuper, Singh-Manoux, Bartley, and Marmot (2004) used a survey item enquiring about an individual's control in the home that had been answered on a six-point scale. The item was "At home, I feel I have control over what happens in most situations" (p. 1503), and participants could choose from six response options ranging from "strongly disagree" to "strongly agree". Chandola et al. (2004, p. 1503) explain that, because most participants endorsed "moderately agree" and "strongly agree" they made the decision to dichotomise the variable into either "low control" (participants endorsing "strongly disagree", "moderately disagree", "slightly disagree", and "slightly agree") or "high control" (participants endorsing "moderately agree" and "strongly agree"). Constructing the variable in this way had subsequent effects on the analyses that were conducted. For Chandola et al. (2004) to proceed as they did, we reasoned that there must have been important meta-method assumptions that enabled them to justify and reconcile the fact that participants endorsing "slightly agree" were regarded as being more similar to participants endorsing "strongly *disagree*" than they were to participants who endorsed "moderately *agree*". Given that this study was one piece of work to better understand the incidence of CHD, this seemed like an important decision to make.

Gilbert (2016) asserts that, partly due to the different ways in which income inequity is measured, the degree of income inequity in the United States (US), and the implications of whatever trend exists, is disputed. A currently unanswered question, for example, is the extent to which income inequity would be affected by a monetised value of leisure time (Gilbert, 2016). Also, decisions about whether or not capital gains, such as wealth derived from owning property, are included in the calculation of income can influence rates of income inequity (Gilbert, 2016). Gilbert (2016) also demonstrates some of the problems in relying on the Gini coefficient as a commonly used measure of income inequity at a national level, when making international comparisons. Moreover, the appropriateness of measures such as Gross National Product (GNP) and Gross Domestic Product (GDP) has been questioned because they might not capture the things that are considered important for a healthy and contented life (Marmot, 2015). Hickel (2017), for example, highlights Bhutan's rejection of GDP and adoption of Gross National Happiness as its measure of social progress. Marmot (2015, p. 290) refers to Robert F. Kennedy's famous speech in which Kennedy instructs us that:

> *… the gross national product does not allow for the health of our children, the quality of their education or the joy of their play. It does not include the beauty of our poetry or the strength of our marriages, the intelligence of our public debate or the integrity of our public officials. It measures neither our wit nor our courage, neither our wisdom nor our learning, neither our compassion nor our devotion to our country, it measures everything in short, except that which makes life worthwhile.*[1]

Measurement is also important when one seeks to understand the way in which income inequity generates stress through social comparisons. How, for example, should the reference group against which comparisons are made, be formed (Gilbert, 2016)? In Chapter 1 we discussed evidence suggesting that, to the extent people compare themselves to others at all, it is people they are similar to on the social ladder who are chosen as the comparator (Wilkinson & Pickett, 2018). In the same vein, Gilbert (2016, p. 69) questions whether "middle-class elementary school teachers in El Paso, Texas, for example, compare their incomes primarily to those of their coworkers, neighbors, the oil barons within the state, Wall Street bankers across the country, Silicon Valley CEOs in California, insurance salesmen in Manhattan, the Mexican workers just across the Rio Grande, or the income of their fathers and siblings?". He considers

[1] https://en.wikipedia.org/wiki/Robert_F._Kennedy%27s_remarks_at_the_University_of_Kansas.

that it is not very likely that these teachers might become despondent "by the thought that Mark Zuckerberg is now on a yacht somewhere in the Mediterranean" as they make their way to work (Gilbert, 2016, p. 70). Gilbert's (2016) point is that there is no clear reason why we should expect all the teachers in El Paso to have the same reference comparison group. The importance of the individuality of people's expectations will be a theme to which we return. The deeply personalised nature of individual expectations is especially important to dwell on for our purposes because Gilbert (2016, p. 70) asserts that to suggest that our personal security, satisfaction, and self-esteem all hinge on where our "household income is positioned relative to a nebulous group of others exemplifies a narrow materialistic assessment of human nature which denies the diverse motives, ambitions, desires, and beliefs that animate people's lives". Gilbert (2016) is eloquently expressing here the point we made in Chapter 1 in relation to our misgivings about widespread and seriously troubling concerns of status and financial gulfs. Gilbert (2016) casts further doubt on the assertion that individual stress is ignited by national levels of income inequity using empirical observations. Japan, for example, has one of the lowest levels of income inequity among developed nations, but also one of the most stressful work environments (Gilbert, 2016).

The way in which studies are designed and conducted can decisively influence the results that are obtained. For instance, Gilbert (2016) points out that what appears to be a relationship between levels of income inequity and rates of teenage births in cross-sectional research disappears when research is conducted longitudinally. He argues, in fact, that "an existing body of longitudinal research offers persuasive evidence refuting the alleged effects of income inequity" (Gilbert, 2016, p. 75). According to Gilbert (2016, p. 76), no-one yet has been able to build a sustained "accumulation of impartial scientific findings" to support the link between income inequity and social problems. Yang, Matthews, and Park (2017) also refer to the importance of the way in which research is planned. Their findings do not support a link between income inequity and mortality, and they suggest the reason that cross-sectional designs do report such a link is because the effects of time are ignored. Whether a researcher chooses a longitudinal or cross-sectional design, therefore, might be determined, at least in part, by the ideological and political meta-method beliefs regarding the results they wish to produce (McIntyre, 2019).

Decisions about which countries to include in international comparisons can also influence the results that are obtained, as can a reliance on the concept of statistical significance as the benchmark of authority. Gilbert (2016) highlights a specific example in which Wilkinson and Pickett (2010) report a relationship between homicide and income inequity. Figure 10.2 in Wilkinson and Pickett (2010) is Fig. 5.1 in Gilbert (2016). Gilbert (2016) explains that, in this particular instance, the US is an extreme outlier and it is only by including it in the analysis that the relationship between homicide and income inequity reaches statistical significance for this collection of countries. If the US is omitted from the analysis, a defensible decision statistically speaking because of its extreme position relative to the other countries, the relationship is no longer statistically significant (Gilbert, 2016). We will have more comments to make about the concept of statistical significance in Chapter 6. At this point, however, it is once again important to highlight McIntyre's (2019) admonishment of the influence of ideological and political beliefs in the results that are reported.

It is also important to be clear about the correspondence between descriptions of results, and the way in which those results were actually produced. Wilkinson and Pickett (2018), for example, state that there is "a substantial body of research showing how well-being and satisfaction with our own pay depends substantially on how it compares with other people's pay" (p. 9), and they provide two references to support this statement. One of those references is a study by Luttmer (2004) who insists, among many claims, that "individuals with richer neighbors report being less happy" (p. 13). Earlier in the report he explains more specifically that "An increase in neighbors' earnings and a similarly sized decrease in own income each lead to a reduction in happiness of about the same order of magnitude" (Luttmer, 2004, p. 3).

When considering Wilkinson and Pickett's (2018) position, along with Luttmer's (2004) original assertion, we assumed that Luttmer (2004) had arrived at this result by assessing the relationship between an individual's happiness and how that individual's income compared with the income of the individual's neighbour. We imagined that what Wilkinson and Pickett (2018) and Luttmer (2004) were communicating was something like the following scenario:

> *During a neighbourly summer barbecue one Sunday afternoon, Frank learns, in a casual conversation with Ahmed who lives across the hedge, that Ahmed earns approximately £3700.00 a month. Frank is really despondent about this because he earns £3200.00 a month, and he knows, based on the presence of the car in the driveway, that he goes to work earlier than Ahmed, and is home later, almost every day.*

Actually, Luttmer's (2004) research finding was quite different from what we had imagined.

Luttmer's (2004) data regarding individual happiness were extracted from two waves (1987–1988 and 1992–1994) of the National Survey of Families and Households. Although the questionnaires were not identical in both waves, Luttmer (2004) considered it appropriate to treat the data as one panel of approximately 10,000 individuals. Individual happiness was assessed on a seven-point scale with one defined as "very unhappy" and seven defined as "very happy" (with no intermediary indicators such as "moderately happy" or "slightly unhappy") in answer to: "Next are some questions about how you see yourself and your life. First taking things all together, how would you say things are these days?" (p. 11). We won't address here how reasonable it might be to assume that a question such as this is accessing people's happiness, but it might be pertinent to point out that this could be regarded as another influential meta-method assumption or the consequence of ideological beliefs. The data used for "Neighbour's income" were even more interesting. Luttmer (2004) obtained data from something called the Public Use Microdata Area (PUMA). According to Luttmer (2004, p. 12), "PUMAs consist of neighborhoods, towns or counties aggregated up, or subdivided, until they contain at least 100,000 inhabitants". In Luttmer's (2004) study, the PUMAs that were included averaged approximately 150,000 people. Luttmer (2004) explains obtaining the measure of neighbour's earnings this way "Average annual earnings in each PUMA are estimated by applying national earnings by industry, occupation and year from the Current Population Survey to the industry and occupation mix of that PUMA from the 1990 Census five percent Public Use Micro Sample" (p. 3) and "The 1990 Census microdata are used to estimate the 3-digit industry × 3-digit occupation composition of each PUMA, which is later used to predict PUMA earnings" (p. 12). The logarithm of this prediction of earnings was then used in the regression analysis.

Luttmer's (2004) construction of the variable of individual income was based on data obtained in the same survey that self-reports of happiness were obtained and is explained as "a set of individual-specific controls that include a number of proxies for income as well as basic demographics" (p. 10), "I average the values of the individual level variables for the main respondent and his or her spouse, and enter those as a single observation in the regression. I thus do not exploit intrahousehold level variation, but this does not matter since the main explanatory variables of interest (neighbors' earnings and own household income) do not vary within households" (p. 11), and "The main income variable is log household income while log value of the home and a dummy for being a renter may also proxy for own income" (p. 12). Table 2.1 depicts these various components and how they relate to some of the reporting that has occurred.

Prior to explaining his approach, Luttmer (2004, p. 7) summarises the results by explaining that "a very basic linear OLS regression with self-reported happiness (on a 1-7 scale) as the outcome variable yields a coefficient of 0.20 (s.e. of 0.014) on log own household income and a coefficient of -0.20 (s.e. of 0.04) on log average per capita income in one's locality (PUMA)". For this analysis then, happiness increased with increases in an individual's household income and decreased with the average income within the individual's locality of approximately 150,000 "neighbours" (or, to be more precise, happiness increased according to changes in the logarithm of these variables). Luttmer (2004) provides the baseline regression equation that produced the main result on page 10. By substituting the actual coefficients for the beta symbols Luttmer (2004) used and ignoring subscripts, the equation is:

$$\text{Happiness} = -0.20(\text{Neighbour's income}) + 0.20(\text{Own household income}) \\ [+\text{a term related to the particular wave of the survey} \\ \text{these data came from} + \text{an error term}]$$

If we just focus on the main variables—which are the variables Luttmer (2004) and others report—some simple algebra produces:

$$\text{Happiness} = 0.20(\text{Own income} - \text{Neighbour's income})$$

The importance and influence of Luttmer's (2004) work should not be underestimated. The title of the article is "Neighbors as negatives:

Table 2.1 Reported statements and data sources used to understand the relationship between happiness and income relative to neighbour's income

Reported Relationship and Source	Components	Data Sources		
		Happiness	**Neighbour's Income**	**Own Income**
• An increase in neighbours' earnings and a similarly sized decrease in own income each lead to a reduction in happiness of about the same order of magnitude; • individuals with richer neighbours report being less happy ○ *Luttmer, 2004* • ... a substantial body of research showing how well-being and satisfaction with our own pay depends substantially on how it compares with other people's pay ○ *Wilkinson & Pickett, 2018*	• Happiness • Neighbour's Income • Own Income	Answers to the question "Next are some questions about how you see yourself and your life. First taking things all together, how would you say things are these days?" on a 7-point scale from 1 (very unhappy) to 7 (very happy) with no defined points in between.	Average annual earnings in each PUMA are estimated by applying national earnings by industry, occupation and year from the Current Population Survey to the industry and occupation mix of that PUMA from the 1990 Census five percent Public Use Micro Sample.	The main income variable is log household income (I average the values of the individual level variables for the main respondent and his or her spouse, and enter those as a single observation in the regression) while log value of the home and a dummy for being a renter may also proxy for own income.

Relative earnings and well-being". It was first published in 2004 in the Harvard University John F. Kennedy School of Government Faculty Research Working Paper Series, and published the following year in the *Quarterly Journal of Economics* where, according to a Google Scholar search on 30 September 2020 it has had 2459 citations. We do not want to give the impression that we are criticising, demeaning, or dismissing this work. And although we have gone into some detail, our primary point and take-home message is to highlight that, sometimes the way research is reported, might give a different impression from the research that was actually conducted.

Seeking Conceptual Clarity

The longer we continued to study the literature, the more we wondered if part of the existing disagreement might have arisen from a lack of conceptual clarity regarding even fundamental ideas. Johnston (2014), for example, reminds us that inequity is much broader than income inequity and includes access and opportunity. Income, however, is easier to measure than access or opportunity (Johnston, 2014). Yet opportunity might be important to understand since increasing equity, and creating greater equity of opportunity, could enhance a nation's productivity (Stiglitz, 2012). Whereas some authors use the terms "access" and "opportunity", Marmot (2015) refers to "capabilities" and suggests that relative inequity in income translates to absolute inequity in capabilities. Capabilities, according to Marmot (2015, p. 43), are "your freedom to be and do".

Bartley (2017) also reminds us that those countries with less income inequity tend to also have better provisions in areas such as health, education, housing, and transport which would enhance the access and opportunities of citizens of those countries. In practical terms, therefore, the most important consideration regarding income inequity is the impact it has on people's lives (Gilbert, 2016). Some authors use the term "income distribution" rather than "income inequity" which may be helpful in directing attention to the way in which resources are shared. Furthermore, the concept of income distribution provides policymakers with a way of improving the psychosocial well-being of whole populations (Wilkinson & Pickett, 2010).

It may also be significant that unequal societies are more competitive and less cooperative than more equal societies (Bartley, 2017). There may need to be greater clarity, therefore, regarding human activities such as cooperation and competition along with characteristics such as trust and community affiliation. Gilbert (2016) points out that such things as trust and a sense of fairness are "states of mind that are difficult to separate from the context in which they are experienced" (p. 80).

Bartley (2017) also appears concerned to clarify another area of confusion. She emphasises that the studies which examine the differences in health between states or countries with unequal income are not actually addressing *health inequity*. Health inequity exists between groups of individuals *within* a single society, not between populations in different geopolitical units. This conceptual opaqueness is reflected in methodological characteristics of studies because some variables, such as life expectancy and murder rates, are aggregates of individual-level variables (Babones, 2008), whereas income inequity is an ecological-level variable (Babones, 2008; Pickett & Wilkinson, 2015).

Causation is another topic in which there is a substantial lack of coherence. Marmot (2015), suggests that health inequities arise through material, psychosocial, and political disempowerment. Similarly, the position of the OECD (2011) is that education and health make the greatest contributions to reducing inequities. Pickett and Wilkinson (2015), on the other hand, conducted a literature review within an epidemiological causal framework, and report that the body of evidence provides support for the satisfaction of major causal criteria with regard to the influence of income inequity on health. This, of course, makes the *a priori* assumption that the epidemiological approach to causation is the most appropriate way to understand relationships between a thing such as health and the factors that may or may not influence it. Perhaps this is another indication of the influence of meta-method ideologies and beliefs.

Even if we accept that income inequity causes poor population health outcomes, we are still left with the question of what to do about it, and, surely, to answer that question, we must understand the nature of the emergence of income inequity. Income inequity is far from inevitable or universal. Its very existence relies on particular economic and political factors. Marmot's (2015) notion of the "causes of the causes" may be appropriate here. Wilkinson and Pickett (2010), in fact, assert that income inequity is an indicator of the degree of social stratification of a society, so, even if we were to follow the causal line of reasoning, is it actually social stratification that should be considered causal of poor population health? It may be the structural causes of inequities that are important to identify and address (Solar & Irwin, 2010) to influence inequity as it manifests in different spheres of social living.

The existing lack of conceptual clarity leads to further questions about other important matters, such as the extent to which distinctions between different types of inequities are actually defensible. Inequities such as income inequity, health inequity, social inequity, inequity of opportunity, and educational inequity are commonly discussed. Is there just *inequity*? Does health inequity seem like it is at the end of some proposed linear causal chain simply because health problems related to inequity take longer to manifest than other sorts of inequities? It will require many years of experiencing educational, income, and social inequities, for example, before coronary heart disease (CHD) appears. Are conditions such as CHD, however, just part of the complete inequity package?

Is a central issue with all inequity nothing more complex than fairness (OECD, 2008)? Are the current political and economic decisions that have enabled the creation of staggering fortunes by the very few, a constant affront to a sense of social justice by many? Starmans et al. (2017) make exactly this point. They argue that there is no evidence to indicate that people are perturbed by economic inequity per se. What bothers people is economic unfairness. A lot of research, however, confuses inequity with unfairness (Starmans et al., 2017). Or, is teasing apart equity and fairness thinking far too much like scientists and academics for the general population? Could we be asking the same kinds of questions about unfairness that we currently ask of inequity? Do most people just want to get through the day by dealing with those things that are directly in front of them at close range?

The importance of the degree to which people are able to function ideally on a day-to-day basis is well recognised, with inequity of *opportunity* considered to be at the core of problems of health inequities (Anand, 2002). Crombie, Irvine, Elliott, and Wallace (2005) also link health inequities with the opportunities people have to improve their physical and social environment, which highlights the importance, not only of opportunities, but also of the interaction of individuals with their environments. The OECD (2008) report recommends that governments should focus on creating equity of opportunities. As others have suggested, the OECD (2008) report also advances the idea that people are willing to accept an *inequity* in income and wealth as long as there is an *equity* of opportunity. Huber et al. (2011) also draw attention to the link between health and the opportunities people have as they interact with their environments. Mackenbach (2017) includes an inequity of opportunity for people to change their social position as one of the reasons for social inequity persisting over time. As with other matters in this area, though, "equity of opportunity" has been another devilishly difficult concept to define that seems to incorporate themes of fairness and control as well as social trust, capabilities, individual perspectives, and the interplay between individuals and their environments. Gilbert's (2016) point about fairness being a state of mind that is difficult to extract from the context in which that mind is embedded is especially relevant here. Johnston (2014) also reminds us that "opportunity" is much harder to measure than, for example, health outcomes. Have pragmatic decisions, therefore, driven a focus on health inequity as much as conceptual and theoretical decisions? Once again, meta-methods seem useful to contemplate here.

The discussion of mechanisms is an area in which there is a large degree of imprecise and inconsistent descriptions. It is difficult to discern, in fact, the way in which a mechanism is conceptualised in the inequity literature. Table 2.2 depicts some of the ways in which the mechanism term has been used in this field. The variety of information provided in the table perhaps obviates the need for any further explanation.

Table 2.2 Terms and descriptions of mechanisms from the health inequity literature along with their sources

Source	Mechanisms
Babones, 2008	Inequity-income-health transmission mechanism; income
Barr et al., 2016	The causal mechanism that connects X and Y; causal mechanisms of a policy's impact
Bartley, 2017	Psycho-neuro-endocrine mechanisms
Beckfield et al., 2015	Welfare state (mediator); three institution mechanisms – redistribution, compression, and mediation
Breznau & Hommerich, 2019	the state
Chandola et al., 2004	Demand overload mechanism; power mechanism; "control at home" as a psychosocial mechanism

(continued)

Table 2.2 (continued)

Source	Mechanisms
Clouston et al., 2016	Risk-factor mechanisms – e.g., smoking cessation, exercise, access to life-saving cancer screening; three meta-mechanisms – spillovers, habitus, and institutional processing; health behaviors
Collins et al., 2015	Psycho-social mechanisms of shame and social comparison; material mechanisms – access to both individual/household resources and public resources (schools, health, social care)
Costa-Lopes et al., 2013	Legitimation a mediating mechanism
Curran & Mahutga, 2018	Two types of mechanisms – psychosocial factors such as status comparison; material resources such as health infrastructure; intervening mechanisms include low social status, underinvestment in public goods, erosion of social cohesion and trust; causal mechanisms; neomaterial mechanisms – neomaterial processes – less economic and administrative capacity, less robust political institutions, minimum resources necessary to obtain adequate health-care; democracy and stability as mechanisms
Diderichsen et al., 2001	Mechanisms of society and mechanisms of human biology; physiological mechanisms; four main mechanisms (also called four conceptual mechanisms) – social stratification, differential exposure, differential susceptibility (also called "differential vulnerability"), and differential consequences
Elliott et al., 2016	Individual strength of character
Gilbert, 2016	The modern welfare state evolved as a social mechanism, According to Clark, the mechanism that conveys social status across generations is not inherited privilege per se but the innate talent inherited from parents, which is nurtured by the transmission of family norms, values, and investments in education and other beneficial activities; many parents in the United States would recoil at the idea of universal child care as a mechanism through which the state aims to neutralize the family's impact on the cognitive development of their offspring; To preserve the plan's financial stability without changing the contribution rate, a balancing mechanism is built into the indexed rate of return. This mechanism is set to automatically reduce the rate return if the pension's liabilities become greater than its assets; when the automatic balancing mechanism was triggered for the first time in 2010, the accounting rules mandated a sudden drop of 4.6 percent in the average pension.
Haack & Sieweke, 2018	Two major mechanisms of income inequity legitimation – adaptation and replacement (the authors note that "the same mechanisms may work in the opposite direction in other contexts").

(continued)

Table 2.2 (continued)

Source	Mechanisms
Hickel, 2017	"abusive transfer pricing" a mechanism that multinational companies use to steal money from developing countries by shifting profits illegally between their own subsidiaries in different countries; monitoring mechanisms; the basic mechanism of profit – the elite simply relied on the fact that the competitive pressures of the labour market (and the market in leases) would increase workers' productivity at a much higher rate than the one at which their wages increased; price- and wage- fixing mechanisms; two basic mechanisms for debt repayment – developing countries had to redirect all their existing cash flows and assets towards debt services and countries that were subject to structural adjustment programmes were forced to radically deregulate their economies; debt became a powerful mechanism for pushing neoliberalism around the world; debt relief has become a mechanism to impose further structural adjustment; enforcement mechanism; a mechanism for policing decisions that are made; investor-state dispute mechanisms; investor-state arbitration mechanism; investor-state dispute settlement mechanisms; three mechanisms of plunder – tax evasion, land grabbing, and climate change
Kragten & Rozer, 2017	Psychosocial and institutional mechanisms
Mackenbach, 2017	Behavioural mechanisms
Marmot, 2015	Having little control over your life is central to the mechanism by which the social environment influences health; biological mechanisms; Scott Matsumoto speculated that the cohesive nature of Japanese culture was a powerful mechanism for reducing stress; we made a virtue of necessity and recommended that countries set up mechanisms to "translate" our recommendations in a form suitable for that country; free-market mechanisms produce better outcomes than heavy-handed and restrictive state regulation; the autonomic nervous system is an essential part of the body's fight-or-flight mechanism; work can influence health by the obvious mechanism of money; one obvious mechanism is through unemployment; there is not a well-developed mechanism for enforcing global working standards
Marmot & Brunner, 2005	Specific biological mechanisms that account for social inequities in cardiovascular disease and diabetes; specific psychosocial, behavioural, and pathophysiological processes – including neuroendocrine, inflammatory, and haemostatic mechanisms

(continued)

Table 2.2 (continued)

Source	Mechanisms
Muntaner et al., 2015	Exploitation mechanism; relational class mechanisms; social mechanisms of exploitation and domination; mechanism-based explanations; context-mechanism-outcome; causal mechanisms
Patel et al., 2018	A possible mechanism proposed for this association was that inequity impacts negatively on social cohesion and capital, and increase chronic stress, placing individuals at a heightened risk of schizophrenia; two mechanisms proposed at the neighbourhood level – social comparison or status anxiety hypotheses, social capital hypothesis
Pickett & Wilkinson, 2015	Causal mechanisms; mediating mechanism
Rothstein & Uslaner, 2005	Feedback mechanisms; causal mechanisms
Rozer et al., 2016	Compositional mechanisms (compositional features and compositional arguments are also mentioned in the same paragraph)
Scambler & Scambler, 2015	Causal mechanisms
Schneider, 2019	Subjective social status is an important psychological mechanism; self-perceptions of social status posited as a key psychological mechanism; a key mechanism through which income inequity contributes to lower status perception is social comparison; important mechanisms are social comparisons and value formation processes; subjective social status a key mechanism (also called a potential mechanism)
Smith et al., 2016	Individual strength of character is stress as a mechanism; causal mechanism
Smith & Schrecker, 2015	Micro-scale mechanisms
Solar & Unwin, 2010	Mechanisms stratify health outcomes – social position; power; "context" is broadly defined to include all social and political mechanisms that generate, configure and maintain social hierarchies, including the labour market; the educational system; political institutions and other cultural and societal values; structural mechanisms are those that generate stratification and social class divisions in the society and that define individual socioeconomic position within hierarchies of power, prestige, and access to resources; the most important structural stratifiers and their proxy indicators include: income, education, occupation, social class, gender, race/ethnicity; social mechanisms; possible mechanisms – nutrition, infection or stress; the main social pathways and mechanisms through which social determinants affect people's health can usefully be seen through three perspectives: (1) "social selection", or social mobility; (2) "social causation"; and (3) life course perspectives; The mechanisms that play a role in stratifying health outcomes operate in the following manner

(continued)

Table 2.2 (continued)

Source	Mechanisms
	• Social contexts create social stratification and assign individuals to different social positions; • Social stratification in turn engenders differential exposure to health-damaging conditions and differential vulnerability, in terms of health conditions and material resource availability; • Social stratification likewise determines differential consequences of ill health for more and less advantaged groups (including economic and social consequences, as well differential health outcomes per se); and • Social mechanisms. The mechanisms through which income could affect health are: • Buying access to better quality material resources such as food and shelter; • Allowing access to services, which may improve health directly (such as health services, leisure activities) or indirectly (such as education); • Fostering self esteem and social standing by providing the outward material characteristics relevant to participation in society; and • Health selection (also referred to as "reverse causality") may also be considered as income level can be affected by health status. General mechanisms that may explain the association between occupation and health-related outcomes are: occupation is strongly related to income; occupations reflect social standing; occupations may reflect social networks; occupation may also reflect specific toxic environmental or work exposures. Social class provides an explicit relational mechanism (property, management) that explains how economic inequities are generated and how they may affect health. As an inherently relational variable, class is able to provide greater understanding of the mechanisms associated with the social production of health inequities. The structural mechanisms that shape social hierarchies, according to these key stratifiers, are the root cause of inequities in health. Together, context, structural mechanisms and socioeconomic position constitute the social determinants of health inequities, whose effect is to give rise to an inequitable distribution of health, well-being and disease across social groups.

(continued)

Table 2.2 (continued)

Source	Mechanisms
	Overcrowding can plausibly affect health outcomes through a number of different mechanisms: overcrowded households are often households with few economic resources and there may also be a direct effect on health through facilitation of the spread of infectious diseases.
	The unequal distribution of these intermediary factors (associated with differences in exposure and vulnerability to health-compromising conditions, as well as with differential consequences of ill-health) constitutes the primary mechanism through which socioeconomic position generates health inequities.
	The communitarian approach defines social capital as a psychosocial mechanism.
	The diagram also highlights the reverse or feedback effects through which illness may affect individual social position, and widely prevalent diseases may affect key social, economic and political institutions.
	Socioeconomic inequities in health can, in fact, be partly explained by the "feedback" effect of health on socioeconomic position, e.g. when someone experiences a drop in income because of a work-induced disability or the medical costs associated with major illness.
	The whole set of "feedback" mechanisms just described is brought together under the heading of "differential social, economic and health consequences". We have included the impact of social position on these mechanisms, indicating that path with an arrow.
	The fundamental mechanisms that produce and maintain (but that can also reduce or mitigate effect) this stratification include: governance; the education system; labour market structures; and redistributive welfare state policies (or their absence).
	The structural mechanisms that shape social hierarchies, according to key stratifiers, are the root cause of health inequities.
Steptoe et al., 2002	Impaired recovery may reflect heightened allostatic load and constitute a mechanism through which low socioeconomic status enhances cardiovascular disease risk.
Stiglitz, 2012	Traditional adjustment mechanisms; traditional economic mechanisms; economic mechanisms; globalization, if managed for the 1 percent, provides a mechanism that simultaneously facilitates tax avoidance and imposes pressures that give the 1 percent the upper hand not just in bargaining within a firm; market mechanisms; a payment mechanism; bankruptcy legislation was used as a legal mechanism; we have the technology to create an efficient electronics payment mechanism

(continued)

Table 2.2 (continued)

Source	Mechanisms
Tracy et al., 2018	Causal mechanisms
Vernon et al., 2015	Control mechanism
Wilkinson & Pickett, 2010	Powerful mechanisms which make people sensitive to inequity; if the link is causal it implies that there must be a mechanism. The search for a mechanism led to the discovery that social relationships (as measured by social cohesion, trust, involvement in community life and low levels of violence) are better in more equal societies; market mechanisms; very explicit mechanisms were used to demonstrate the intent that all would have a share of future wealth
Wilkinson & Pickett, 2018	A small developmental advantage becomes magnified through classroom interactions in just the same way as small genetic differences in one or other skill or ability can become magnified by practice as people select and are selected by their environment. The same mechanism explains why more than twice as many professional hockey players are born in the first three months of the year than in the last three months. It is likely that small genetic advantages in one or other activity have such an influence on individual development because we get pleasure from doing what we are best at relative to others ... A mechanism of this kind, which pushes siblings to differentiate themselves from each other, would explain why some research suggests that siblings are not more alike than random pairs of the population. We now have a clearer understanding of where individual differences in ability come from and how children's differing circumstances affect the subsequent development of their cognitive capacity. Income and status differences are, as we have seen, at the heart of these processes at the level of the individual, but bigger income differences also reduce educational outcomes across whole societies. We have seen something of the mechanisms behind these processes, how they affect the vast majority of the population, and why they damage those at the bottom most. The theory that economic inequity has damaging social consequences has indeed led to many testable predictions, covering outcomes and causal mechanisms which have been repeatedly confirmed.

Concluding Comments and Common Themes

You will, of course, draw your own conclusions from the material we have presented and critiqued; even to the extent of how accurately and impartially we have represented the available information. We certainly do not claim to have completed an exhaustive review. Rather, our aim was to capture the main themes, concepts, ideas, and points of contention that currently exist in this literature. Wherever some of the ideas or claims raise queries or doubts for you, we would encourage you to investigate the original sources as we have done.

While much of the empirical work regarding health inequity has produced interesting findings, the findings are also limited in scope and applicability. The acknowledgement of both the conceptually and empirically fractured state of the field, and the questions that still require answers, suggests that pausing to consider a new perspective might not be time wasted. On the contrary, our sense from the available information is that a good many of the current ideas are pointing in a consistent direction. A map, or robust understanding of the nature of that which is being studied, might permit many of these apparently antagonistic ideas to be organised into a more coherent picture.

As we conclude our overview of the health inequity literature, we are aware that we have consistently emphasised the disagreement that appears to us to characterise this domain. Despite this emphasis, it is not the disagreement that we are bothered by. On the contrary, we concur with McIntyre (2019, p. 298) that dissension can be healthy in ongoing research if researchers focus on the best way to investigate important questions "not whether the answers produced are politically acceptable". We do consider, however, that the inequity arena might have reached somewhat of an impasse regarding current theorising and methodologies.

Although we were no closer to understanding why, based on the current body of knowledge, inequity should *necessarily* be the problem it is portrayed to be, nor why the large amount of effort directed to researching it and understanding it had not revealed widespread, systematic solutions, we were encouraged by the themes we had identified. In particular, it seemed to us that terms such as fairness, equity, opportunity, control, trust, empowerment, and capability, were all hinting at something important, but currently unrecognised. Our tentative, yet informed suggestion, is that the theoretical, or meta-method framework we outline in the next chapter might provide the light to reveal both existing conceptual linkages that currently seem invisible, as well as the very beginnings of a path to somewhere new.

References

Anand, S. (2002). The concern for equity in health. *Journal of Epidemiology and Community Health, 56*(7), 485–487.

Babones, S. J. (2008). Income inequality and population health: Correlation and causality. *Social Science and Medicine, 66,* 1614–1626.

Barr, B., Bambra, C., & Smith, K. E. (2016). For the good of the cause: Generating evidence to inform social policies that reduce health inequalities. In K. E. Smith, S. Hill, & C. Bambra (Eds.), *Health inequalities: Critical perspectives* (pp. 252–263). Oxford: Oxford University Press.

Bartley, M. (2017). *Health inequality: An introduction to concepts, theories and methods* (2nd ed.). Cambridge: Polity Press.

Beckfield, J., Bambra, C., Eikemo, T. A., Huijts, T., McNamara, C., & Wendt, C. (2015). An institutional theory of welfare state effects on the distribution of population health. *Social Theory & Health, 13*(3–4), 227–244. https://doi.org/10.1057/sth.2015.19.

Blazquez-Fernandez, C., Cantarero-Prieto, D., & Pascual-Saez, M. (2018). Does rising income inequality reduce life expectancy? New evidence for 26 European countries (1995–2014). *Global Economic Review: Perspectives on East Asian Economies and Industries, 47*(4), 464–479. https://doi.org/10.1080/1226508X.2018.1526098.

Breznau, N., & Hommerich, C. (2019). The limits of inequality: Public support for social policy across rich democracies. *International Journal of Social Welfare, 28,* 138–151.

Carey, T. A., Huddy, V., & Griffiths, R. (2019). To Mix or Not To Mix? A meta-method approach to rethinking evaluation practices for improved effectiveness and efficiency of psychological therapies illustrated with the application of Perceptual Control Theory. *Frontiers in Psychology, 10,* 1445.

Chandola, T., Kuper, H., Singh-Manoux, A., Bartley, M., & Marmot, M. (2004). The effect of control at home on CHD events in the Whitehall II study: Gender differences in psychosocial domestic pathways to social inequalities in CHD. *Social Science & Medicine, 58,* 1501–1509.

Crombie, I. K., Irvine, L., Elliott, L., & Wallace, H. (2005). *Closing the health inequalities gap: An international perspective.* Copenhagen: WHO Regional Office for Europe. Accessed on 4 March 2021 from https://apps.who.int/iris/bitstream/handle/10665/107680/E87934.pdf?sequence=1&isAllowed=y.

Clouston, S. A. P., Rubin, M. S., Phelan, J. C., & Link, B. G. (2016). A social history of disease: Contextualizing the rise and fall of social inequalities in cause-specific mortality. *Demography, 53,* 1631–1656. https://doi.org/10.1007/s13524-106-0495-5.

Collins, C., McCrory, M., Mackenzie, M., & McCartney, G. (2015). Social theory and health inequalities: Critical realism and a transformative activist stance? *Social Theory & Health, 13*(3–4), 377–396.

Costa-Lopes, R., Dovidio, J. F., Pereira, C. R., & Jost, J. T. (2013). Social psychological perspectives on the legitimation of social inequality: Past, present and future. *European Journal of Social Psychology, 43,* 229–237.

Curran, M., & Mahutga, M. C. (2018). Income inequality and population health: A global gradient? *Journal of Health and Social Behavior, 59*(4), 536–553.

Diderichsen, F., Evans, T., & Whitehead, M. (2001). The social basis for disparities in health. In T. Evans, M. Whitehead, F. Diderichsen, A. Bhuiya, & M. Wirth (Eds.), *Challenging inequities in health: From ethics to action* (pp. 12–23). New York: Oxford University Press.

Elliott, E., Popay, J., & Williams, G. (2016). Knowledge of the everyday: Confronting the causes of inequalities. In K. E. Smith, S. Hill, & C. Bambra (Eds.), *Health inequalities: Critical perspectives* (pp. 222–237). Oxford: Oxford University Press.

Freeman Anderson, K., Bjorklund, E., & Rambotti, S. (2019). Income inequality and chronic health conditions: A multilevel analysis of the U.S. States. *Sociological Focus, 52*(1), 65–85. https://doi.org/10.1080/00380237.2018.1484251.

Gilbert, N. (2016). *Never enough: Capitalism and the progressive spirit*. Oxford: Oxford University Press.

Haack, P., & Sieweke, J. (2018). The legitimacy of inequality: Integrating the perspectives of system justification and social judgment. *Journal of Management Studies, 55*(3), 486–516. https://doi.org/10.1111/joms.12323.

Hickel, J. (2017). *The divide: A brief guide to global inequality and its solutions*. London: Penguin Random House.

Huber, M., Knottnerus, J. A., Green, L., van der Horst, H., Jadad, A. R., Kromhout, D., … Smid, H. (2011). How should we define health? *BMJ, 343,* d4163. https://doi.org/10.1136/bmj.d4163.

Johnston, D. C. (2014). Introduction. In D. C. Johnston (Ed.), *Divided: The perils of our growing inequality* (pp. i–vii). New York: The New Press.

Kragten, N., & Rozer, J. (2017). The income inequality hypothesis revisited: Assessing the hypothesis using four methodological approaches. *Social Indicators Research, 131,* 1015–1033.

Luttmer, E. F. P. (2004). *Neighbors as negatives: Relative earnings and well-being* (KSG Working Paper No. RWP04-029). Accessed 12 September 2020. https://papers.ssrn.com/sol3/papers.cfm?abstract_id=571824.

Mackenbach, J. P. (2017). Persistence of social inequalities in modern welfare states: Explanation of a paradox. *Scandinavian Journal of Public Health, 45,* 113–120.

Marmot, M. (2015). *The health gap: The challenge of an unequal world.* London: Bloomsbury.

Marmot, M., & Brunner, E. (2005). Cohort profile: The Whitehall II study. *International Journal of Epidemiology, 34,* 251–256.

McIntyre, L. (2019). *The scientific attitude: Defending science from denial, fraud, and pseudoscience.* Cambridge, MA: The MIT Press.

Muntaner, C., Ng, E., Chung, H., & Prins, S. J. (2015). Two decades of Neo-Marxist class analysis and health inequalities: A critical reconstruction. *Social Theory & Health, 13*(3–4), 267–287. https://doi.org/10.1057/sth.2015.17.

OECD. (2008). *Growing unequal? Income distribution and poverty in OECD countries.* Paris: OECD Publishing. Accessed 12 September 2020. https://www.oecd.org/els/soc/growingunequalincomedistributionandpovertyinoecdcountries.htm.

OECD. (2011). *Divided we stand: Why inequality keeps rising.* Paris: OECD Publishing. Accessed 12 September 2020. https://www.oecd.org/els/soc/dividedwestandwhyinequalitykeepsrising.htm.

Patel, V., Burns, J. K., Dhingra, M., Tarver, L., Kohrt, B. A., & Lund, C. (2018). Income inequality and depression: A systematic review and meta-analysis of the association and a scoping review of mechanisms. *World Psychiatry, 17*(1), 76–89.

Pickett, K. E., & Wilkinson, R. G. (2015). Income inequality and health: A causal review. *Social Science and Medicine, 128,* 316–326.

Rothstein, B., & Uslaner, E. M. (2005). All for all: Equality, corruption, and social trust. *World Politics, 58*(1), 41–72.

Rozer, J., Kraaykamp, G., & Huijts, T. (2016). National income inequality and self-rated health: The differing impact of individual social trust across 89 countries. *European Societies, 18*(3), 245–263. https://doi.org/10.1080/14616696.2016.1153697.

Scambler, G., & Scambler, S. (2015). Theorizing health inequalities: The untapped potential of dialectical critical realism. *Society Theory & Health, 13*(3–4), 340–354.

Schneider, S. M. (2019). Why income inequality is dissatisfying—Perceptions of social status and the inequality-satisfaction link in Europe. *European Sociological Review, 35*(3), 409–430. https://doi.org/10.1093/esr/jcz003.

Smith, K. E., & Schrecker, T. (2015). Theorising health inequalities: Introduction to a double special issue. *Social Theory & Health, 13*(3–4), 219–226. https://doi.org/10.1057/sth.2015.25.
Smith, K. E., Bambra, C., & Hill, S. (2016). Background and introduction: UK experiences of health inequalities. In K. E. Smith, S. Hill, & C. Bambra (Eds.), *Health inequalities: Critical perspectives* (pp. 1–21). Oxford: Oxford University Press.
Solar, O., & Irwin, A. (2010). *A conceptual framework for action on the social determinants of health. Social Determinants of Health Discussion Paper 2 (Policy and Practice)*. Geneva: World Health Organization. Accessed 12 September 2020. https://www.who.int/sdhconference/resources/ConceptualframeworkforactiononSDH_eng.pdf.
Starmans, C., Sheskin, M., & Bloom, P. (2017). Why people prefer unequal societies. *Nature Human Behavior, 1*(0082). https://doi.org/10.1038/s41562-017-0082.
Steptoe, A., Feldman, P. J., Kunz, S., Owen, N., Willemsen, G., & Marmot, M. (2002). Stress responsivity and socioeconomic status: A mechanism for increased cardiovascular disease risk? *European Heart Journal, 23,* 1757–1763.
Stiglitz, J. E. (2012). *The price of inequality*. London: Penguin.
Tracy, M., Cerda, M., & Keyes, K. M. (2018). Agent-based modelling in public health: Current applications and future directions. *Annual Review of Public Health, 39,* 77–94.
Vernon, D., Lowe, R., Thill, S., & Ziemke, T. (2015). Embodied cognition and circular causality: On the role of constitutive autonomy in the reciprocal coupling of perception and action. *Frontiers in Psychology, 6,* 1660.
Wilkinson, R., & Pickett, K. (2010). *The spirit level: Why equality is better for everyone*. London: Penguin Books.
Wilkinson, R., & Pickett, K. (2018). *The Inner level: How more equal societies reduce stress, restore sanity and improve everyone's well-being*. London: Penguin Random House.
Yang, T.-C., Matthews, S. A., & Park, K. (2017). Looking through a different lens: Examining the inequality-mortality association in U.S. counties using spatial panel models.

CHAPTER 3

Inequity Through a Different Lens: An Introduction to Perceptual Control Theory

Facts are stubborn things, and whatever may be our wishes, our inclinations, or the dictums of our passions, they cannot alter the state of facts and evidence. John Adams

In the previous two chapters we described our impressions of the state of the health inequity literature, as we encountered it, while we hunted for answers to the questions of why inequity is *necessarily* the problem it is portrayed to be, and why it has been so impervious to remedies. The field, in general, seems to be a gallimaufry of ideas, concepts, methodologies, standards, and explanations. We think this is a problem because, *if* there is an issue to be addressed, and *if* the issue is important enough that it compromises successful social living, then anything less than a unified, coherent approach will jeopardise effective resolution of the issue.

In this chapter we will expose and explain the important meta-methods that provided the lens through which we considered the material we were consuming. These meta-methods all exist within the one overarching theoretical framework, which we will do our best to describe succinctly. It is this framework and these meta-methods that, we believe, could provide a perspective to open the inequity field to important new, more productive, lines of enquiry. The information in this chapter might also provide a context for our seemingly irascible attitude towards the existing body of knowledge.

T. A. Carey et al., *Deconstructing Health Inequity*,
https://doi.org/10.1007/978-3-030-68053-4_3

Let's Start at the Very Beginning

Perhaps the first meta-method assumption that we need to share is that we think, in order to understand how to fix something, it is important to understand the "working-just-fine" state of that something. To put it another way, in order to repair an entity that is broken, in fact, to even know whether or not the entity *is* broken and needs repair, it is essential to be familiar with the unbroken form of the entity. How does the entity in question function when it is working ideally?

We would attribute, for example, much of the vagueness in the mental health field to the fact that the "normal" state of psychological functioning has never been unambiguously defined. The entire mental health realm, in fact, has proceeded to research and treat mental *disorder* without ever describing what mental *order* might be. A consequence of this ambiguity is that what is and is not classified as mental disorder appears to depend largely on the authority of the classifier.

For a discipline to describe itself as a legitimate science, it seems to us that precision and accuracy should be two of the highest standards. It is attitude, not method, that defines activity as scientific (McIntyre, 2019). As Table 3.1 indicates, four possible scenarios exist with regard to the combination of accuracy and precision. Just suppose, a good friend of ours, the enigmatic Claudette Twahira, lives at 12 Chalcot Square, Primrose Hill, London. We could tell you that Claudette lives in England, which would be accurate, but not very precise. Or, we could tell you that Claudette lives at 23 George Street, Pialba, Hervey Bay, Queensland, Australia which would be very precise but not accurate. We could

Table 3.1 The relationship between accuracy and precision as important priorities for science

		Accuracy	
		High	Low
Precision	High	Physical Sciences	
	Low		Behavioural Sciences (?)

also tell you that Claudette lived in Brattleboro, Vermont in the United States which would not be accurate or precise. The address of 12 Chalcot Square, Primrose Hill, London, however, is both accurate *and* precise. The explanatory power of the physical sciences can, perhaps, be explained by the penchant in those areas for high standards of both precision and accuracy. In some ways, it seems that the life sciences might have adopted statistical significance as their benchmark of rigour rather than precision and accuracy. And there you have it—another meta-method has just snuck out. We think the rigorous expectations of the physical sciences are norms to which the life sciences should aspire. Because the subject matter of the life sciences, though, is different from the subject matter of the physical sciences, it's likely that, in many cases, we'll need *different* approaches to achieve the *same* impeccable standards of rigour. McIntyre (2019, p. 304) comments that "the study of human behavior needs to be based on theories and explanations that are relentlessly tested against what we have learned through experiment and observation".

While we're setting the context for the information we'll provide, you should understand that another meta-method standard of ours is a conviction that theories worth paying attention to are theories of some*thing*. And the more that something is an actual, tangible, physical phenomenon, the greater is the opportunity for a precise and accurate theoretical explanation to be developed and rigorously tested. We would contend that much of the imprecision in the field of behavioural science is because an accurate and precise definition of behaviour has never been unequivocally established. We think there is a very good reason for that which we will explain below. To introduce you to the lens which has become our window to the world, we will begin with a physical demonstration of a phenomenon.

A simple activity will demonstrate the phenomenon we want to share with you and also help focus the following discussion. The activity is a tracking task that can be undertaken by anyone who chooses to follow this link:

https://www.mindreadings.com/ControlDemo/BasicTrack.html.

If you visit this site, you'll see, at the top of the screen, the rectangular frame with two short vertical bars depicted in Fig. 3.1. The top vertical bar remains stationary throughout the activity, but the bottom vertical bar moves backwards and forwards in a straight line across the screen staying within the frame of the rectangle. In this activity, the upper vertical bar is called the target and the lower vertical bar is called the cursor.

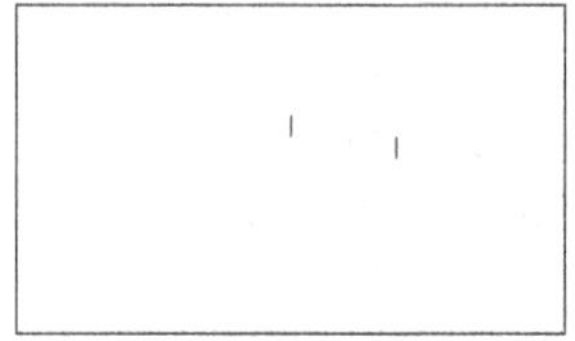

Fig. 3.1 Appearance of the computer screen prior to the commencement of the tracking task showing the target and the cursor

Immediately beneath the rectangle is a little box with the words "New Run" in it. If you click on that box, you can use the mouse to control the position of the cursor.

The task is relatively simple. Once "New Run" is clicked, the mouse can be used to keep the cursor aligned with the target. The activity lasts for approximately 30 seconds. At the end of 30 seconds, results are provided. If no action is taken with the mouse, the cursor moves across the screen for 30 seconds according to one of several randomly selected (selected by the computer programme not the person completing the activity) computer-generated movement patterns. By using the mouse, however, it is possible, in fact quite easy, to counteract this programmed movement to keep the cursor lined up with the target.

This straightforward tracking activity is useful and instructive in a number of ways. Because it is conducted on a computer, data are able to be recorded to quantify the relationships established by the activity. Three important relationships can be discerned. There is a relationship between the movement of the mouse and the position of the cursor. There is also a relationship between the movement of the mouse and the unseen and unpredictable force that is simultaneously acting upon the cursor. Finally, we can also consider the relationship between the position of the cursor and the unseen and unpredictable movement pattern of the computer program.

When a person completes this activity, and we would strongly encourage you to do that before you read on, the position of the cursor relative to the target represents the goal the person adopts. The movement of the mouse is the person's actions (behaviour) and the computer-generated movement pattern is the extraneous, unknown, and unpredictable environmental force. The process of keeping the cursor in a particular relationship with the target is the phenomenon we'll be exploring. The tracking task is useful and instructive because it demonstrates some of the important principles of *all* behaviour. Actually, it's probably more accurate and precise to say that the activity demonstrates a different way of thinking *about* behaviour but we won't digress to explain *that* detail just yet.

Another important feature of this activity is that once the 30 second task has been completed, a model is immediately applied to the data as a way of explaining the behaviour by testing the model. The test of the model is the degree to which the model accurately and precisely matches the behaviour of the mouse movements. Model fitting of this kind is rare in the behavioural sciences but the *method du jour* of the physical sciences. Because of the model fitting feature of this activity, we can refer to this task as an "experiment".

Before commencing the experiment, it might be useful to articulate some of what we expect to find. Table 3.2 indicates what reasonable hypotheses might be based on existing knowledge in the behavioural sciences. Given current, conventional understanding of the nature of goals and actions, for example, it would be reasonable to expect that the experiment will demonstrate a strong relationship between these two variables. Similarly, perhaps we would predict a weak relationship between a person's actions and the unseen, unknown, and unpredictable environmental forces of the computer-generated movement pattern. We might also predict a weak relationship between a person's goal and those same environmental forces.

The results of six experiments, in terms of the plots of the data for each relationship, are provided in Fig. 3.2. Because of the amount of data collected, the relationships can also be accurately and precisely quantified

Table 3.2 Predicted relationships, based on conventional psychological knowledge, between a person's goal, the person's actions, and environmental effects

	Cursor (Goal)	**Mouse (Actions)**	**Disturbance (Environment)**
Cursor (Goal)		Strong relationship	Weak relationship
Mouse (Actions)	Strong relationship		Weak relationship
Disturbance (Environment)	Weak relationship	Weak relationship	

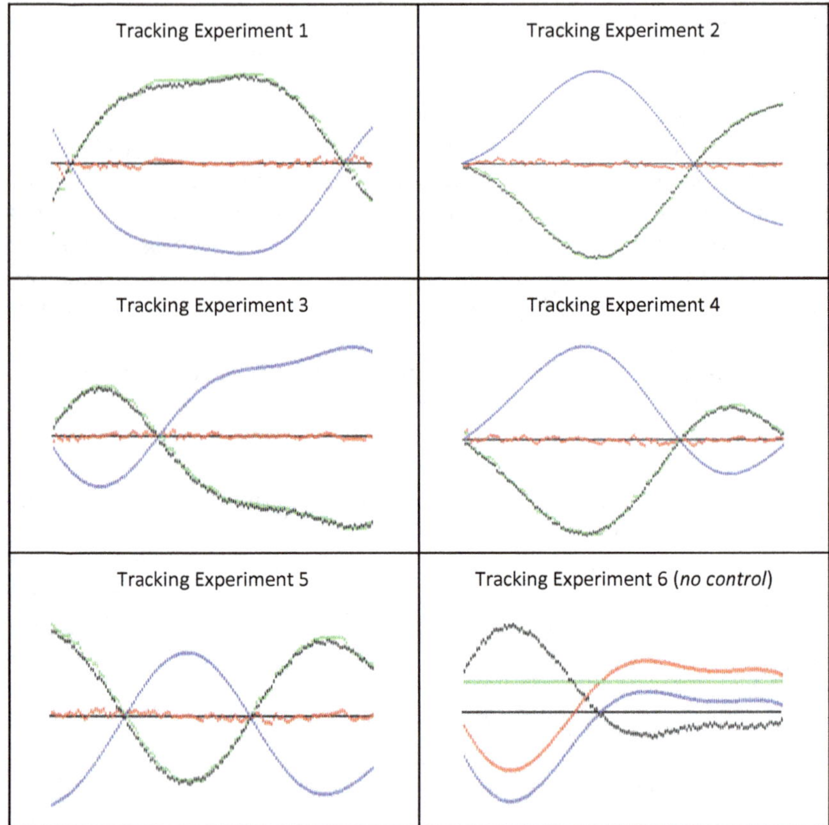

Fig. 3.2 Results of six tracking experiments performed by the same person (Tim) with the sixth experiment involving no control. Red = Cursor; green = Mouse; blue = Disturbance; black = Model

(see Table 3.3). In Fig. 3.2, the first five plots were experiments in which Tim (first author) used the mouse to keep the cursor aligned with the target. The sixth plot is included only for illustrative purposes. Experiment 6 is the scenario described earlier in which the mouse is inactive, so the movement of the cursor in this experiment was determined entirely by the computer program. In the plots in Fig. 3.2, the green line is a record of the position of the mouse (Tim's actions) during the 30 seconds of the experiment, the red line is a record of the position of the cursor relative

Table 3.3 Correlations between each of the pairs of variables over six trials of the tracking experiment: Cursor and Mouse (Goal and Actions); Mouse and Disturbance (Actions and Environment), Cursor and Disturbance (Goal and Environment); and Mouse and Model (Actions and Test of Assumptions)

Tracking Experiment	Quantified Relationships			
	C & M (G & A)	M & D (A & E)	C & D (G & E)	M & Mdl (A & ToA)
1	0.183	-0.996	-0.092	0.995
2	-0.134	-0.999	0.177	0.999
3	0.153	-0.999	-0.117	0.999
4	0.045	-0.999	0.009	0.998
5	0.092	-0.998	-0.033	0.998
6 *(No control)*	0.000	0.000	1.000	0.000

C = Cursor; M = Mouse; D = Disturbance; Mdl = Model; G = Goal; A = Actions; E = Environment; ToA = Test of Assumptions

to the target (Tim's goal), and the blue line is a record of the movement pattern generated by the computer. The black line is a record of the model's explanation of the actions in the experiment. Experiment 6 demonstrates that when the mouse is stationary, the movement of the cursor is the same as the movement pattern generated by the computer.

Inspection of the plots illustrates what the quantitative results confirm. Perhaps the first thing to notice is the remarkable symmetry between the green and the blue lines (behaviour and environmental disturbance). This beautiful pattern is an autograph of the phenomenon we are demonstrating and explaining. It could well be nature's most spectacular accomplishment.

In Experiments 1–5, the mouse movements and the unpredictable computer-generated movement pattern are in an almost perfect inverse relationship. This is accomplished even though the mouse movements are different in every experiment and the computer-generated movement pattern was completely unknown to Tim in every experiment. The correlation coefficients for this relationship are in the column labelled "M & D" in Table 3.3. They range from −0.996 to −0.999. It can be deduced from a brief study of the plots that the position of the cursor (the red line) *at every point in time* was *jointly determined* by the position of the mouse, and the value of the computer-generated movement pattern. That is, if the value of the computer-generated movement pattern was −30 pixels, the mouse would be in such a position that it represented somewhere in the very near vicinity of 30 pixels on the computer screen, giving a value for the cursor of approximately 0 and, thereby, keeping it aligned with the target. So, it was *never* just Tim's response (actions), *nor* the stimulus of the computer-generated movement pattern that *caused* the cursor to be where it was. It was the *combined* effects of both of these forces *simultaneously* and *constantly*. As will be explained below, this analysis of causality is diametrically opposed to the way in which causality seems to be typically conceptualised in the health inequity domain as a linear process.

The other striking result from these experiments that seems apparent from Fig. 3.2 is the *lack* of a relationship between Tim's goal and the actions used to achieve that goal. Again, inspection of the correlation coefficients in Table 3.3 confirms this assumption. The coefficients in the column labelled "C & M" range from −0.134 to 0.183. Given the amount of data used to calculate these coefficients, these results would be highly statistically significant yet the lack of any sort of useful relationship is blatantly obvious. The third especially noteworthy result is the startling fit between the actions and the model. The coefficients in the column in Table 3.3 labelled "M & Mdl" range from 0.995 to 0.999. This is an unparalleled result for model precision and accuracy in the behavioural sciences.

The predictions that were recorded in Table 3.2, therefore, are quite different from the actual results obtained. Table 3.4 provides a revised version of Table 3.2 in which the results that were obtained, rather than predicted, are provided. From the standpoint of the way in which behaviour is conventionally understood, these results are practically incomprehensible. The results indicate that there is no discernible relationship between a person's goal (target) and the actions the person takes to achieve that goal. Yet, there is an extremely strong, almost perfect relationship, between a person's actions and unseen, unknown, and unpredictable environmental forces. This activity demonstrates, and we will explain in more detail below, that for humans, and indeed all living things, to achieve the results they intend, they *do not* control their behaviour. On the contrary, they allow their behaviour to *vary* according

Table 3.4 Actual relationships revealed by the tracking experiments demonstrate a weak relationship between a person's goal and the actions used to achieve that goal and a very strong relationship between the person's actions and unseen and unpredictable environmental effects

	Cursor (Goal)	**Mouse (Action)**	**Disturbance (Environment)**
Cursor (Goal)		Weak relationship	Weak relationship
Mouse (Action)	Weak relationship		Strong relationship
Disturbance (Environment)	Weak relationship	Strong relationship	

to the vagaries of their immediate environment, so that the *outcomes* they intend *are* controlled.

The Ubiquitous Phenomenon of Control

The explanation that accurately and precisely accounts for these results, and makes sense of the notion that we do not control behaviour, is known as Perceptual Control Theory (PCT; Powers, 1973, 2005). As the name suggests, PCT is a theory about control, and about perceptual control in particular. Use of the term "perceptual" distinguishes organic, autonomous control from the control of inanimate devices such as household heating thermostats and the cruise control systems in cars.

While the term "control" is commonly used in a wide variety of contexts, in PCT it has a precise and accurate definition. Control is regarded as a phenomenon of nature. "Control is a real, objective phenomenon that involves the production of consistent results under varying environmental conditions" (Marken, 1988, p. 196). It is the specific phenomenon of stability in the face of variability (Marken, 1988, p. 197). Control is the red line (goal or target) despite the presence of the blue line (environmental disturbance). Powers (2005, p. 296) defines control as "Achievement and maintenance of a preselected perceptual state in the controlling system, through actions on the environment that also cancel the effects of disturbances". Further perusal of Experiments 1–5 in Fig. 3.2 provides a visual demonstration of this definition with the red line illustrating the preselected perceptual state, the green line illustrating the actions on the environment, and the blue line illustrating the disturbances. The symmetry between the green and the blue lines illustrates the way in which the actions cancel the effects of the disturbances to maintain a stable goal state continually.

The plots in Fig. 3.2 are the map of a new and exciting territory. They provide a visual representation, perhaps, of why the idea of "balance" seems to resonate so strongly with so many people across so many different areas. PCT explains that the current quest of attempting to establish a reliable relationship between goals and actions is the equivalent of trying to spin straw into gold. We need a different perspective if we intend to strike gold within the behavioural sciences in terms of a precise and accurate understanding of the conduct of living things.

Control, then, is what we regard as the "normal" state of affairs for entities that live. In fact, the phenomenon of control provides the ideal description of the "normal" state of affairs for creatures that live. "The business of turning parts of the environment into yourself and defending yourself against the inevitable disintegration – that is what control is all about. That is life. Rocks don't do that. Every cell in an organism like us does that. Every gene in a creature like us does that. Every complex self-replicating molecule in every living creature does that" (Bourbon, personal communication, 20 November 2000).

Living things, therefore, function effectively when they can achieve and maintain the preselected perceptual states that are important to them, despite environmental effects that would otherwise alter these states. Any assessment of disruptions to functioning should only be made relative to the preselected perceptual states of the individual concerned. A "successful career" or a "happy marriage" could be preselected perceptual states. A "finishing time under two hours" for a half marathon could be another preselected perceptual state. A "decaf soy latte", "newspaper in bed on a Sunday morning", "phone calls from friends on my birthday", and "feeling calm and safe in public" might all be preselected states that people maintain through their actions on their environments. Are "fairness" and "equity" some other preselected perceptual states that are important to many people? We still weren't sure of the answer to *that* question, but we did think it might be an important question to entertain.

The process of control, and indeed the importance of control for living creatures, has been acknowledged for some time in isolated pockets of scientific enquiry. Homeostasis, for example, is well established as the process that maintains our body temperature within a stable range. Marks (2018) is a contemporary psychological scientist who has, independently, recognised the fundamental importance of homeostasis. Marks (2018, p. 2) maintains that, "all behaviour is an expression of homeostasis". He has built a general theory of behaviour around this neglected but indispensable concept which he maintains could unify the field and "take a few measured steps towards advancing Psychology as a natural science" (p. X). Such an ambition is entirely consistent with the spirit of this book.

Homeostasis is a control process. Fung (2016) describes homeostasis as the defining characteristic of life on earth. Coincidentally, PCT theorists view control as being synonymous with life. Bourbon (1995, p. 151) explains that "Life is control – an uninterrupted process of specifying, creating, and maintaining – a process in which all that is not essential is free to change, preventing change in what is essential". Marmot (personal communication June 13, 2018) is equally unambiguous in his view regarding the centrality of control to the social determinants of health. As another example, Collins, McCrory, Mackenzie, and McCartney (2015) describe agency as the essence of being human. From a PCT perspective, "agency" is one of the many pseudonyms the phenomenon of control has acquired.

The PCT point of view is that control is the underlying process whenever any aspect of living is contemplated. Bourbon (personal communication, 20 November 2000), for example, explains it this way:

> *... the perceptual hierarchy exists for one purpose – that it serves as a means by which intrinsic physiological reference conditions can be created and maintained. That is what comes first, and last, and all the time in between. We think that the self-replicating molecules, like those in DNA, are control systems, complete with their equivalents of reference signals that specify which "perceptions" of molecular shape, or of chemical states, they will "sense". On this construal, genes are not "commands" for what we will become, but they are control systems that control for certain molecular states; all of the rest that happens is in a way one big side-effect of control at the biochemical level. If that is so, then it must be the case that, more often than not, creatures like us, with perceptual hierarchies like ours, end up being good environments for DNA to achieve its own control.*

A statement such as this communicates a sentiment that is remarkably similar to Gribbin's (1998, p. 116) assertion that "Biologists have an aphorism that 'a hen is the egg's way of making more eggs'. In the same way, a human being is simply the genes' way of making more copies of themselves".

Invariant Laws Will Not Be Discovered Through the Study of Variability

The plots from Experiments 1–5 in Fig. 3.2 provide numerous lessons. As the first five plots reveal, actions were different on every occasion. This is an example of the variability that is a central feature of research activity in the behavioural sciences. PCT, on the other hand, is a study or explanation of *invariance*, which is the red line in the plots from Experiments 1–5. Thus, another meta-method understanding of ours has been brought to light. It is our contention that the accuracy, precision, and explanatory power of the physical sciences is due, in large part, to their propensity for studying invariant properties of the natural world (Carey & Mansell, 2009; Carey, Huddy, & Griffiths, 2019). The behavioural sciences, however, have focussed on the study of *variability*. Scientific laws will never be established through a better understanding of variability. Powers (1990, p. 24) expresses clearly and potently what might be regarded as the general motivation behind the behavioural sciences' dogged crusade to tame the variable aspects of our social and personal landscape:

> *It is commonly assumed that statistical generalizations found from empirical studies of human or animal behavior reflect more detailed underlying processes. When we lack understanding of detailed mechanisms, all we can do is look at general relationships between dependent and independent variables; presumably, these relationships will someday be proven to arise from underlying biological mechanisms of behavior. When we finally understand those mechanisms, goes the assumption, we will see that they provide the reasons for the empirical findings.*

Mechanisms and Models

In Chapter 2 we described the way in which mechanisms are presented in the inequity literature. In this field, the term "mechanism" refers to a hodgpodge of concepts, processes, and systems. Referring to such a potpourri of things as mechanisms is again, for us, out of step with standards of accuracy and precision. More importantly, however, is the fact that conceptual and statistical mechanisms will not lead to the discovery of actual, physical mechanisms. Once again, Powers's (1990, p. 31) wisdom has been, for us, instructive in extending and clarifying the views he provided in the passage above:

> *... it is not possible to proceed in the other direction, that is, from the statistical study to the underlying mechanism. It is not true that a relationship observed statistically using many subjects (even identically organized subjects) necessarily reflects any relationship that would be found through understanding the underlying mechanisms. The hope that statistical studies will eventually lead us to understanding of mechanisms is in vain. It is more likely that statistical studies will lead us to deduce the wrong mechanisms. We have only one way of learning about underlying mechanisms and that is to find models of them that work.*

Powers (1990) indicates here his strong preference for models that work. PCT is, fundamentally, a model of how control works. Models of this ilk provide a much more exacting test of one's assumptions than statistical or conceptual models. It was, for us, illuminating to learn about the way in which Powers (1990, p. 24) approached the task of modelling:

> *In contrast to the method of statistical generalization, the method of modeling begins by analyzing an individual behaving system. First, the system is broken down into actual or proposed components, each of which can be described as a simple input-output relationship. Then the equations describing each component are solved as a simultaneous system to predict the individual's behavior, given the actions of any independent outside influences. The calculated behavior is compared against the actual behavior with those same influences acting. The difference between the model's behavior and the real behavior provides a basis for systematically revising the hypothetical components of the model (the known components, of course, remain the same) until its calculated behavior is in accord with observation. The method of modeling is the basis for most procedures in the physical sciences. Generalizations come afterward, not first. There is, in fact, almost no use of statistical generalization in the most successful sciences. The focus is on constructing and improving models.*

The way in which Powers (1990) describes his approach to modelling has strong parallels with the way in which Galileo has been described as conducting his scientific activity. Taylor (2003, p. 17) explains that "Often as part of his desire to understand how something worked, Galileo built himself a model. He was essentially a hands-on person rather than a theorist and found that the act of constructing the model could be as valuable as observing it working when it came to understanding the principle behind a natural phenomenon". Powers's (1990) attitude also resonates strongly with Feynman's famous pronouncement that "If it disagrees with experiment, it's wrong". Standards such as this have, as yet, failed to infiltrate the behavioural sciences in any comprehensive way.

Considering Causality

Thus, it might be apparent that another of our meta-methods is that building physical models that work should be prioritised above the construction of statistical or conceptual models. Moreover, the evidence generated from models that work should be regarded as superior, by orders of magnitude, to the evidence provided by models that are statistical or conceptual. One of the lessons from the construction of these models, that has profound implications for the behavioural sciences generally, and the inequity field in particular, is the way in which causality is understood. Powers (2005) was able to demonstrate that, for living things, the notion of linear cause and effect is incomplete and misleading. When seeking to understand the activity of living things, circular, rather than linear, causality is the appropriate model to adopt. Actually, the recognition of circular rather than linear causality is quite an old idea despite how little appreciated it still is. Dewey (1896, p. 363), over 120 years ago, advised that, even with something as fundamental as a reflex arc:

> *What we have, is a circuit, not an arc or broken segment of a circle. This circuit is more truly termed organic than reflex, because the motor response determines the stimulus, just as truly as sensory stimulus determines movement. Indeed, the movement is only for the sake of determining the stimulus, of fixing what kind of a stimulus it is, of interpreting it.*

Powers (2008, pp. 17–18) explains that with entities that are alive, organisation is critical:

> *One of the principles adopted by biology and other life sciences has been that organisms are made of matter and therefore obey all the laws that govern the*

behavior of matter. While this is true, it is also untrue. It's not true that they obey ONLY the laws that govern the behavior of matter. ... Laws that apply to lumps of material do not necessarily apply when the material is organized in ways other than lumps. If you analyze an airplane chemically or physically, it will prove to be made of materials that can't, in their raw form, fly. Yet they can be organized to fly.

The principle that organisms obey the laws of matter has therefore been more misleading than helpful. It has led to thinking that the same causal laws apply to living systems as to nonliving ones. While that is true at a certain level of observation-you can cause a mouse to fly by throwing it into the air-it is not true at any higher level. You can't cause a mouse to jump into the air by itself if it doesn't want to.

Zimring (2019, p. 342) provides a contemporary endorsement of Powers's (2008) position by explaining that "The current view is that living things are made of the same elements as nonliving things, and it is simply the way that they are combined, and not some life force, that gives rise to organic chemicals".

But Doesn't Everyone Already Know All This?

In some ways, we wouldn't be surprised if, after having got this far in the chapter, you are wondering what all the hullabaloo is about. Isn't this information we already know? It is certainly true that references to control and related concepts are liberally peppered throughout the health inequity literature. We have already mentioned Marmot's firm stance with regard to control. At times, Marmot (2015) appears to use the terms "control" and "empowerment" interchangeably. He considers having little control over one's life as fundamental to the processes by which the social environment influences one's health. He is by no means alone in his recognition of the importance of control.

Costa-Lopes, Dovidio, Pereira, and Jost (2013) highlight the importance of justice standards in establishing important factors such as control and predictability. Wilkinson and Pickett (2010) describe the importance of control in the workplace. Wilkinson and Pickett (2018) discuss a range of different benefits in both the workplace and people's lives generally when they have greater control. Smith, Bambra, and Hill (2016) suggest that much of the relevant research conducted in the United Kingdom (UK) confirms the contribution of control to health outcomes. Control has been described as being strongly linked to ill health (Diderichsen, Evans, & Whitehead, 2001), and there appears to be a general acceptance that when stress is experienced in social situations it is due to a lack of control (Williams & Collins, 1995). Burns (2014), in fact, views control as central to understanding health inequity.

There are also less direct references throughout the literature. Despite their more indirect nature, however, the essence of control is still clear. Gilbert (2016) advises that the practical significance of income inequity can only be ascertained in terms of how it impacts on people's lives. From a PCT perspective, it can easily be appreciated that, any impact on a person's life, given that living is a control process, would concern control. Even though Vernon, Lowe, Thill, and Ziemke (2015) use the term "allostasis" they describe a process of achieving goal stability in the midst of uncertain circumstances so this clearly fits within the framework of control. Themes of autonomy and self-determination can also be regularly found in the literature. Similarly, there are frequent references to the importance of freedom (Marmot, 2015) and opportunity (Stiglitz, 2012) in relation to inequity and health.

Even the concept of circular causality is not completely invisible. Solar and Irwin (2010), for example, recognise that the relationship between health and agency is not uni-directional. They suggest that while health promotes agency, agency and freedom also yield better health. Once again, we would regard control as central to the concept of agency. Vernon et al. (2015) also recognise the importance of a departure from linear causality claiming that a reciprocal linking between perceptions and actions is well established.

While the volume of informal recognition indicating the importance of control is definitely encouraging, what is glaringly absent is an explanation of how control works. Our firm conviction is that the work and insights of the researchers mentioned above, as well as the efforts of other contributors to health inequity knowledge who we have not explicitly mentioned, would all benefit by being based on an appreciation of how control works. Richard S. Marken is a prolific PCT scientist whose rigorous work includes the tracking experiment we introduced earlier in this chapter. He explains the contribution of PCT this way (Marken, R. S., email, CSGnet, 12 July 1997):

> *PCT is probably just a more formal and precise formulation of these people's implicit theory of human nature. Understanding this precise formulation can help you do your work better. People were able to shoot cannonballs pretty accurately before Newton came up with the laws of motion because the cannonball shooters understood (implicitly) Newton's third law (action/reaction). But with these laws (which are a theory of motion, like PCT is a theory of behavior) the cannonball shooters could shoot cannon balls even more accurately. With PCT, a therapist is in a position to work more "accurately" than the person without the theory.*

Marken's (1997) point here is important and worth reiterating. It is likely that PCT will only be of interest and benefit to those people who want to do things—research, practice, policy—better. For those researchers, clinicians, professionals, and policymakers who are doing things about as well as they would like, PCT, and in fact the remainder of this book, will probably have little to offer.

In a Nutshell

The meta-method assumptions that direct our attention and guide our work have had a marked effect on the way in which we have digested the health inequity literature. For us, control is the phenomenon of life. On this point, we would extend Fung's (2016) assertion by clarifying that it is negative feedback control that is defining of life on this planet. Negative feedback is as fundamental to control as natural selection is to evolution. In fact, the parallels with evolution are strong. Control is both fact and theory (Marken, 1988). Control (constantly achieving goals in the context of unpredictably varying environments) is a fact like evolution (as evidenced by the fossil record). These facts are explained by PCT through the negative feedback loop and natural selection, respectively (Marken, 1988). To summarise, control is a fact that the theory of negative feedback explains.

The current perspective through which the behavioural sciences views both routine and aberrant conduct needs to be traded for the lens of control.

The normal state of affairs for people is being able to control the things that are important to them. The bustle of living things cannot be divorced from the environments in which they bustle. Whereas, up until now, the study of human behaviour has been, to a very great extent, studied from a third-person, observer perspective, the lesson from PCT is that it is the *first-person* perspective that must be the object of enquiry. We must develop the same unrelenting fixation with preselected perceptual states that we have, until now, maintained on observable behaviour. Behaviour *is* the control of perception and, so, it is the perceptions that must hold our gaze.

PCT has rigorously demonstrated that living things control their perceptual input *not* their motor output (Marken, 2014). As the plots in Fig. 3.2 vividly illustrate, actions vary according to the whims of the environment so that perceptual standards *do not* vary, or vary only according to edicts from within the system. This suggests long-standing and widespread neglect by the behavioural sciences of the most fundamental feature of human activity.

From an understanding of control, important implications can begin to be described. It is not possible, for example, to understand what someone is doing by only observing their actions. It is entirely through an appreciation of people's preselected perceptual states along with the way they experience their current environment that their conduct can be accurately understood. PCT also introduces a very useful relativity consideration into the task of being able to fathom the way in which people are affected by environmental circumstances. Someone will only be troubled, or bothered, or distressed, or traumatised, or experience some other unpleasantness, if the happenings in their environment overwhelm their abilities to act, or otherwise impair their ability to control. This relativity of control explains why the same event will not be similarly traumatising to all people, and the sight of a Palladium Silver Bentley Continental GT sitting in front of the neighbour's garage door will not send all people into downward spirals of debilitating anxiety. PCT explains why "it depends" is such a sensible and accurate way of approaching people, their problems, and the lives they are forging for themselves.

At this point, we had arrived at some preliminary answers to our questions with which, for now, we were satisfied. The answers are:

1. Inequity is *not necessarily* a problem. Compromised control is the problem. Matters such as inequity and unfairness will only be problems to the extent that they indicate or signal compromised control. There can be inequitable situations, however, where people are still able to control the things that are important to them.

and

2. The reason that the problem has been so difficult to address systematically and thoroughly is because we have been scrutinising it through the wrong lens. PCT provides a different, and we would contend, more accurate, more precise, and therefore, ultimately, more useful lens.

By understanding ourselves, other people, and our social systems, from the perspective of control, we will have the opportunity to scale greater heights of understanding and develop solutions that are monumentally more sustainable and comprehensive. A failure to recognise control will make it seem like there are inconsistent and often puzzling results. For the remainder of the book we will describe in more specific details the implications for health inequity, if an understanding of activity as control is adopted and wholeheartedly embraced by researchers, health professionals, and policy and other decision-makers.

References

Bourbon, W. T. (1995). Perceptual control theory. In H. L. Roitblat & J. A. Meyer (Eds.), *Comparative approaches to cognitive science* (pp. 151–172). Cambridge, MA: MIT Press.

Burns, H. (2014). What causes health? *Journal of Royal College of Physicians of Edinburgh, 44,* 103–105.

Carey, T. A., Huddy, V., & Griffiths, R. (2019). To mix or not to mix? A meta-method approach to rethinking evaluation practices for improved effectiveness and efficiency of psychological therapies illustrated with the application of perceptual control theory. *Frontiers in Psychology, 10,* 1445.

Carey, T. A., & Mansell, W. (2009). Show us a behaviour without cognition and we'll show you a rock rolling down a hill. *The Cognitive Behaviour Therapist, 2,* 123–133.

Collins, C., McCrory, M., Mackenzie, M., & McCartney, G. (2015). Social theory and health inequalities: Critical realism and a transformative activist stance? *Social Theory & Health, 13*(3–4), 377–396.

Costa-Lopes, R., Dovidio, J. F., Pereira, C. R., & Jost, J. To. (2013). Social psychological perspectives on the legitimation of social inequality: Past, present and future. *European Journal of Social Psychology, 43,* 229–237.

Dewey, J. (1896). The reflex arc concept in psychology. *The Psychological Review, 3*(4), 357–370.

Diderichsen, F., Evans, T., & Whitehead, M. (2001). The social basis for disparities in health. In T. Evans, M. Whitehead, F. Diderichsen, A. Bhuiya, &

M. Wirth (Eds.), *Challenging inequities in health: From ethics to action* (pp. 12–23). New York: Oxford University Press.

Fung, J. (2016). *The obesity code: Unlocking the secrets of weight loss*. London: Scribe Publications.

Gilbert, N. (2016). *Never enough: Capitalism and the progressive spirit*. Oxford: Oxford University Press.

Gribbin, J. (1998). *Almost everyone's guide to science*. London: Weidenfeld & Nicholson.

Marken, R. S. (1988). The nature of behavior: Control as fact and theory. *Behavioral Science, 33,* 196–206.

Marken, R. S. (2014). *Doing research on purpose: A control theory approach to experimental psychology*. St. Louis, MO: New View.

Marks, D. F. (2018). *A general theory of behaviour*. London: Sage.

Marmot, M. (2015). *The health gap: The challenge of an unequal world*. London: Bloomsbury.

McIntyre, L. (2019). *The scientific attitude: Defending science from denial, fraud, and pseudoscience*. Cambridge, MA: The MIT Press.

Powers, W. T. (1973). *Behavior: The control of perception*. Chicago: Aldine.

Powers, W. T. (1990). Control theory and statistical generalizations. *American Behavioral Scientist, 34*(1), 24–31.

Powers, W. T. (2005). *Behavior: The control of perception* (2nd ed.). New Canaan, CT: Benchmark.

Powers, W. T. (2008). *Living control systems III: The fact of control*. New Canaan, CT: Benchmark.

Smith, K. E., Bambra, C., & Hill, S. (2016). Background and introduction: UK experiences of health inequalities. In K. E. Smith, S. Hill, & C. Bambra (Eds.), *Health inequalities: Critical perspectives* (pp. 1–21). Oxford: Oxford University Press.

Solar, O., & Irwin, A. (2010). *A conceptual framework for action on the social determinants of health*. Social Determinants of Health Discussion Paper 2 (Policy and Practice). Geneva: World Health Organization. Accessed 12 September 2020. https://www.who.int/sdhconference/resources/ConceptualframeworkforactiononSDH_eng.pdf.

Stiglitz, J. E. (2012). *The price of inequality*. London: Penguin.

Taylor, I. (2003). *Galileo: A beginner's guide*. London: Hodder & Stoughton.

Vernon, D., Lowe, R., Thill, S., & Ziemke, T. (2015). Embodied cognition and circular causality: On the role of constitutive autonomy in the reciprocal coupling of perception and action. *Frontiers in Psychology, 6,* 1660.

Wilkinson, R., & Pickett, K. (2018). *The Inner level: How more equal societies reduce stress, restore sanity and improve everyone's well-being*. London: Penguin Random House.

Wilkinson, R., & Pickett, K. (2010). *The spirit level: Why equality is better for everyone*. London: Penguin Books.

Williams, D. R., & Collins, C. (1995). US socioeconomic and racial differences in health: Patterns and explanations. *Annual Review of Sociology, 21,* 349–386.
Zimring, J. C. (2019). *What science is and how it really works*. Cambridge: Cambridge University Press.

CHAPTER 4

Health Through the Lens of Control: A Different Look at Well-Being and Being Well

The habit of an opinion often leads to the complete conviction of its truth, it hides the weaker parts of it, and makes us incapable of accepting the proofs against it. Jons Jacob Berzelius

It seems reasonable to suggest that, if any systematic and sustained improvements in the health and equity arena are going to be achieved, a clear idea of what health is might be a necessary starting point. Currently, health inequity is assessed through apparent indicators of health such as infant mortality and life expectancy (Beckfield et al., 2015; Bezruchka, 2014; Blazquez-Fernandez, Cantarero-Prieto, & Pascual-Saez, 2018). Other indicators include the presence of various diseases and also premature death (Mackenbach, 2017). Despite the way in which health inequity is assessed, there doesn't seem to be any indication that a preference is developing for referring to "life expectancy inequity" or "disease inequity". Instead, the term "health inequity" is used consistently.

So, what is health? Without a precise and accurate definition of what health is, the way in which one decides what a premature death, as opposed to a mature or expected death, might be, is not obvious. Moreover, given that death is a non-negotiable aspect of living, it will always be the case that some people who die, do so without being unhealthy. Of course, whether or not we agree that healthy people can die could depend entirely on the way in which health is defined and understood.

T. A. Carey et al., *Deconstructing Health Inequity*,
https://doi.org/10.1007/978-3-030-68053-4_4

Well then, *if* control is the order of the day for living things, as we're suggesting it is, what does that mean for the way in which we think about health? What is the "compromised control" we mentioned at the end of the last chapter, and why should anyone take notice of it? Is PCT and this control malarkey just a whole lot of blah, blah, blah or is there something worth paying attention to? Is it simply another version of that word substitution game that we often see played in the behavioural sciences which is possible because of the way in which terms and phrases are only vaguely and inadequately defined? Are we conceptually shuffling deckchairs on an inequity Titanic with no substantive improvement appearing over the horizon? Is PCT yet another example of a concept or idea that is all tip and no iceberg? Or maybe this all just sounds like "old hat" or some obvious and common sense thing you already knew about.

If you've managed to arrive at this place in the book, we wouldn't be surprised if one or more of these sentiments is crashing ceaselessly against the inside of your forehead. In this chapter we'll describe our ideas for the contribution control generally, and PCT more specifically, might make for the way in which we understand health and, consequently, health inequity. Our ambition is that, by the time you get to the end of the chapter, we will have provided enough information so that your current pounding is now a soothing but irrepressible urge to know more.

What Is Health?

Despite the apparent ubiquity of the term, and the frequency with which it is discussed in a broad range of contexts, health turns out to be a rather slippery concept to define. So far, no universally accepted definition has emerged regarding what we mean when we refer to or discuss "health". The definition provided in the World Health Organization's (WHO) 1946 Constitution remains its standard. The definition asserts that "Health is a state of complete physical, mental and social well-being and not merely the absence of disease or infirmity" (WHO, 1946). WHO's definition has been recognised as groundbreaking for its time but also criticised for becoming increasingly inadequate (Huber et al., 2011, 2016; Saylor, 2004). How many of us can say that we have truly attained a state of *complete* physical, mental, and social well-being, for example (Huber et al., 2011)?

Developing a clear and precise definition of health is not just an academic exercise. The way in which health is considered has important policy and practice implications for such things as the allocation of resources (Carey, 2017; Saini et al., 2017). Koplan et al. (2009) make the point that, in the area of global health, without a clear definition, it will not be possible to reach agreement on such fundamental issues as what is trying to be achieved, the appropriate approaches to take, and so on. Saini et al. (2017) remind us that many benchmarks for disease thresholds are determined by professional societies, guilds, and committees that often have conflicts of interest due to their relationships with industry. Committees, for example, in which members had numerous links with the pharmaceutical industry, changed the standard for what was considered a safe and appropriate cholesterol level (Moynihan & Cassels, 2005). Moynihan and Cassels (2005) reported that initially 13 million United States (US) citizens were considered to be in need of treatment, however, with subsequent committee decisions, this number swelled to 36 million and then 40 million. In the absence of unambiguous criteria, it becomes impossible to demarcate necessary treatment from overdiagnosis and overmedicalisation with the consequent waste of finite resources.

Without any clear statement about what separates health from disease, or, indeed, whether these constructs are best understood in such dichotomous terms, authorities are given little choice but to base their decisions on opinion rather than evidence. The invented categories of mental disorder, for example, appear or disappear from the American Psychiatric Association's (APA) *Diagnostic and Statistical Manual of Mental Disorders* (APA, 2013) based on the voting trends by members of various committees (Timimi, 2014). Unsurprisingly, the validity of nosological systems used in psychiatry, and the extent to which they accurately describe discrete disease entities, has been deemed questionable (Jablensky, 2016). There have been calls, therefore, for the psychiatric profession to abandon current systems of classification (Hengartner & Lehmann, 2017; Timimi, 2014). Given the unhealthy, indeed corrupt, relationship that has been described between the APA and the pharmaceutical industry (Whitaker & Cosgrove, 2015), determining the condition of psychological and social functioning through a flawed committee voting process can hardly be considered acceptable or scientific.

Some people prefer to avoid attempting to define health at all (Anand, 2002) or defer to the WHO definition mentioned above (e.g. Burns, 2014). Without dwelling on the definition of health, Burns (2014) takes a different approach. He makes some important points relevant to health inequity by considering the factors and conditions that might enkindle health.

Other people have, however, proposed their own suggestions for a definition of health. Although the definitions often vary in terminology and emphasis, we believe it is possible to identify a common thread or theme. In other words, looking through the window of control, we have been able to spot relevant ideas and concepts. It is as though a pigeon has been thrown among the cats. The pigeon is under a blanket so the cats can't see it. They don't know what it is, but they can see it squirming around and they are very sure (as sure as a cat can be) that there is some delectable treat that is waiting for them if they could only figure out how to lift the blanket. We hope this chapter will help in that endeavour.

Fung (2016), who describes homeostasis as the defining feature of life, is perhaps closer to lifting the blanket than many others. Marks (2018) is another who, it appears, may have lifted the blanked. His general theory of behaviour is homeostasis at its core. The term "homeostasis" was first coined by the physiologist Walter Bradford Cannon (1932). It describes the processes through which the physiological conditions that are essential for an organism's survival are maintained in a relatively steady state (Davies, 2016). Homeostasis, for us, is just control by another name. Haack and Sieweke (2018) describe adaptation as being important when considering how health might be defined. Bircher (2005) is another who seems to come close to the concept of control, but then also appears to drift away. According to Bircher (2005), individuals strive to be in control. Health, though, from Bircher's (2005) perspective, is an ongoing state of well-being involving something Bircher (2005) refers to as "potential". Bircher (2005), perhaps, provides a very useful illustration of why and how a robust, functional theory can assist in ensuring that ideas and concepts are parsimonious and consistent. We would argue that, in the absence of accurate and precise definitions, the relationship between health and well-being is not at all straightforward. The term "health" as it is generally used refers to physical health or "being well". People can experience physical health conditions that make them feel unwell, yet still maintain a sense of well-being. Conversely, people can be seriously troubled but be physically healthy. Therefore, well-being and being well are not equivalent (Carey, 2013).

The idea of being able to adapt and manage oneself within our environment is common in the literature discussing definitions of health, as is the notion of a state of equilibrium (Huber et al., 2011). Galderisi, Heinz, Kastrup, Beezhold, and Sartorius (2015) highlight the importance of equilibrium in their efforts to define mental health. They also refer to the pertinence of culture when considering definitions of matters such as these. Saylor (2004), too, recognises the relevance of culture and explains the shortcomings of current conceptualisations of health, as being narrowly focussed on a Western biomedical understanding. Incorporating ideas from other cultures, Saylor (2004) highlights the centrality of a sense of purpose as well as balance, adaptation, and equilibrium. The integration of mind and body is also embedded within ideas and practices from other cultures (Saylor, 2004).

The Australian Aboriginal and Torres Strait Islander cultures provide a specific example of the significance of considering different cultural perspectives. The widely cited current definition of health from an Aboriginal and Torres Strait Islander point of view is “Not just the physical well-being of the individual but the social, emotional, and cultural well-being of the whole community. This is a whole-of-life view and includes the cyclical concept of life-death-life” (National Health Strategy Working Party, 1989, p. x). This definition is a summary statement from a more expanded explanation on the previous page of the National Health Strategy. The information provided is:

> *“Health” to Aboriginal peoples is a matter of determining all aspects of their life, including control over their physical environment, of dignity, of community self-esteem, and of justice. It is not merely a matter of the provision of doctors, hospitals, medicines or the absence of disease and incapacity.*
>
> *Prior to colonisation Aboriginal peoples had control over all aspects of their life. They were able to exercise self-determination in its purest form. They were able to determine their “very-being”, the nature of which ensured their psychological fulfilment and incorporated the cultural, social and spiritual sense.*
>
> *In Aboriginal society there was no word, term or expression for “health” as it is understood as in Western society. It would be difficult from the Aboriginal perception to conceptualise “health” as one aspect of life. The word as it is used in Western society almost defies translation but the nearest translation in an Aboriginal context would probably be a term such as “life is health is life.”*

> *In contemporary terms Aboriginal people are more concerned about the "quality of life". Traditional Aboriginal social systems include a three-dimensional model that provides a blue-print for living. Such a social system is based on inter-relationships between people and land, people and creator beings, and between people, which ideally stipulates inter-dependence within and between each set of relationships.* (National Health Strategy Working Party, 1989, p. ix)

Traditionally, therefore, their equivalents of concepts such as control and self-determination were the ways in which Aboriginal and Torres Strait Islander peoples thought about "health".

An editorial in the Lancet (2009) explicitly emphasises the importance of being able to adapt to one's environment and goes on to explain that this necessarily incorporates an understanding of self-determination. Health as adaptation inevitably means that health will vary from individual to individual, and therefore, health must be defined by the patient, not the doctor (Lancet, 2009). Self-determination is mentioned in other contexts in conjunction with concepts such as agency and goals (Solar & Irwin, 2010). Burns (2014), by drawing on the work of earlier authorities, acknowledges the fundamental nature of adaptation and the consequent unavoidable presence of control. Burns (2014, p. 104) suggests that "If a feeling of being in control of our lives and being able to make decisions for ourselves is an important determinant of how individuals create health" then this understanding should be reflected in public policy.

Even when processes rather than terms are described in the literature, a similar theme of control and equilibrium can be discerned. Bracken (2013) discusses the notion of an ultimate cause in which the state of a healthy cell is tipped, so that it becomes a tumour, or compromises embryological development, or impairs the immune system. Similarly, Marmot (2015) suggests that, psychologically, the times when there is a sense that it is all getting to be too much, are the times when one is not able to control the things that matter.

Through the lens of control, then, all of the different concepts such as agency, homeostasis, purpose, equilibrium, balance, and adaptation are all the cats circling the pigeon of control. To our way of thinking, semantic differences have obscured the fact that these terms are, in fact, all referring to the process of control. If control is the process of living, then health *is* control (Carey, 2016). The phenomenon of control and the explanation of how it works (PCT; Powers, 1973, 2005) provide an elegant framework for incorporating all of the concepts mentioned in this section. Moreover, given the nature of the phenomenon of control, as we will explain below, it easily applies cross-culturally as well as integrating not just mind and body but cell and gene, as well as partnership, family, and community.

Controlling Is a Bio—Psycho—Social Process

The need to understand the interconnectivity between different aspects of human functioning is certainly not new. Engel (1977, 1980), more than four decades ago, suggested that the prevailing model of biomedicine should be replaced by what he termed a biopsychosocial model. McLaren (1998) has pointed out that, despite Engel's (1977, 1980) conviction of the importance of a biopsychosocial model, he never articulated what that model should be. Powers (1973, 2005), however, has provided a model that could be exactly the kind of model to which Engel (1977, 1980) seems to have been referring.

The phenomenon of control, established through the physical mechanism of negative feedback, has been identified at all levels of functioning (Carey, Mansell, & Tai, 2014). Powers (1973, 2005) has described a network of negative feedback control systems which are organised hierarchically so that control at one level is achieved by varying the standard required at the level below. At all levels, exactly the same negative feedback control process occurs, with the difference being the complexity of the perceptual variables that are controlled. At lower levels, simpler perceptions are controlled such as the brightness of light or the correct combination of pitch and rhythm of a favourite melody. At the higher, loftier levels reside perceptions such as principles including honesty, loyalty, or fairness as well as systems concepts such as community or personality.

The hierarchical nature of negative feedback control systems can be appreciated by asking oneself a series of *why* and *how* questions. Asking why questions generally lead a person's awareness to travel to ever higher levels within the perceptual hierarchy, bringing increasingly abstract goals to mind. If you were to ask yourself why you voted for one political party rather than another, for example, your reasons might include the particular values you believe that political party embodies or the kind of society you hope to live in. If, instead, you asked yourself how you voted for your political party of choice, it is likely that you would report a series of more prosaic goals. Walking to the polling booth, for example, or placing an X on the ballot paper next to your chosen candidate. Whether the goals we are considering relate to the creation of a society that we perceive to be just or writing an X on a piece of paper, PCT argues that these events occur through the same process of negative feedback control.

Understanding health as control would promote a more seamless appreciation of the conduct of being human. Marmot (2015), for example, refers to a psychosocial dimension which he suggests can be described as having control over one's life. We have no quarrel with Marmot (2015) on this score, but we would contend that it is not just the psychosocial dimension that contributes to the control people have in their lives. Burns's (2014) comments in terms of a feeling of being in control are also relevant here. Burns (2014) is not the only one to refer to a feeling of being in control or having a sense of control. His comments, though, are very helpful in assisting to illustrate the point we are making here. From our perspective, people don't, in fact, have control *over* their lives. Nor is simply a feeling of being in control the issue that matters. Life *is* control. It is necessary to ***actually*** control important variables. Feelings of being in control can be comforting but they are ultimately useless in terms of maintaining the integrity of an organism in the absence of actual control. Maintaining a steady body temperature or blood glucose level is exactly the same control process as maintaining a steady career progression or a stable friendship group. From this angle, each of these variables, and many more, needs to be controlled for a person to be "healthy".

What Would Thinking About Health in This Way Mean?

Recognising health as control, permits the clarification of important points as well as the refinement of other decisive matters. Saracci (1997) and WHO (2017) are two of many who declare health to be a basic human right. From a health is control perspective, however, health is much more important and fundamental than being relegated the status of a human right. We wouldn't, for example, suggest that homeostasis is a fundamental human right. Control is a property of the way we are designed. Digestion is not a human right. Neuroplasticity is not a human right. Cell regeneration is not a human right. The depolarisation of a neuronal cell membrane would hardly be designated the status of a basic human right. Perhaps if health as control was considered in the same way as digestion or respiration, decision-makers such as politicians and policy writers would think differently about the conditions which allow financial and other resources to be distributed inequitably.

When health is discussed, and especially in Western biomedical contexts, it is frequently imbued with judgemental and prejudicial connotations. It is common to find, for example, references to the "healthy choices" or the "poor health choices" someone might be making, which can easily turn into "victim-blaming". Understanding health as control, however, draws attention to the goal states people are keeping in balance by the way we see them conducting themselves in the world segment we share. The matter of interest then becomes whether or not they are controlling their goal states satisfactorily, with the understanding that "satisfactorily" can only be judged from their perspective. That is, the standard of satisfactory, in the context provided here, only makes sense as a first-person, rather than a third-person, attitude.

The term control, over the years, has also attracted some rather unflattering and negative connotations. An inflexible person who insists on imposing their will on others might be described as a "control freak", for example. A quick Internet search of the term control will return numerous hits for articles with topics like "How to deal with controlling people", or "10 ways to recognise controlling behaviour". What PCT illustrates, however, is that we are all controlling people (Marken & Carey, 2015). Control is an inevitable and immutable phenomenon that is central to defining what it means to be alive.

A critical development in the health as control paradigm would see an elevation of the preferences and perspective of the patient. There is strong evidence that failure to pay appropriate attention to patient preferences has played a decisive role in the rise of the global scourge of inappropriate care, which wastes exorbitant amounts of health funds each year (Saini et al., 2017). The overdiagnosis and overmedicalisation mentioned above are aspects of the occurrence of inappropriate care. The necessity of transforming our current patient-centred model of care into a patient-perspective model of care (Carey, 2017) will be discussed in the penultimate chapter.

Becoming familiar with a health as control way of seeing the world will permit a more accurate understanding of what we regard as behaviour, as well as the way in which different forces, factors, and influences affect each other. In particular, from a control vantage point, there is an imperative to reconsider the way in which we currently approach causality. We will have more to say about causality in the next chapter but, for now, it is important to highlight that the social determinants of health are actually *not* determinants. The social determinants of health (Beckfield et al., 2015; Marmot, 2006; Solar & Irwin, 2010) has been an important campaign for drawing attention to circumstances and conditions that were not, historically, considered the purview of health. By acknowledging that health is control, however, we could develop more accurate and precise ways of understanding the resources people have available to them in any given environment, and the degrees of freedom they have to create lives of their own design. On the other hand, referring to resources, situations, and circumstances as "determinants" situates people as passive objects subject to the whims of their environments, rather than as active agents who are the contemplators and craftsmen of their lives. When an active agents position is absorbed, the necessity and ramifications of considering an equity of opportunity (OECD, 2008) approach might be more readily appreciated. There is no doubt that the environment an individual inhabits has important impacts on their health (Burns, 2014) but an accurate understanding of control would allow a more nuanced appreciation of the way in which the environmental circumstances either impedes or promotes each individual's controlling.

By explicating the workings of the phenomenon of control, more nuanced discussions might be possible regarding the way in which people can achieve more of their goals more of the time. Vernon, Lowe, Thill, and Ziemke (2015) in their discussion of self-determination refer to the degree to which a system establishes its own goals as well as the degree to which the environment of the system does *not* control the system's behaviour. If the system being referred to is a control system, however, Powers (1973, 2005) has demonstrated that while a system's goals are set autonomously, once they have been specified, the behaviour or output of the system is determined *entirely* by the environment. If this point requires clarification, refer back to Experiments 1–5 in the previous chapter and reflect on the meaning of the red, green, and blue lines.

Another important aspect of social living that impacts on health and is related to control, concerns the way in which we structure social relationships. As we suggested earlier, there appears to be evidence to suggest that inequity is related in some way to competition and cooperation. Wilkinson and Pickett (2018) indicate, for example, that more equitable societies are also more cooperative societies. While Wilkinson and Pickett (2018) focus almost exclusively on status competition, PCT (Powers, 1992) explains the problems of competition more pervasively. Mackenbach (2017) appears to concur with this stance by suggesting that social inequity is the outcome of competition. Understanding people as control systems illuminates the problems that competition poses. Competition, from a control systems perspective, represents conflict between systems (Marken & Carey, 2015). Conflict for control systems is *always* detrimental because, for the period of time that conflict exists, control is thwarted. While Kragten and Rozer (2017) propose that unequal societies produce higher levels of competition, from a PCT perspective, we could reason that, in fact, the situation is actually the reverse. We would maintain that control can become compromised through such things as policies promoting competition with consequences of impaired physical, social, and psychological functioning. Taxation policies which favour wealthy people would be an example. Gilbert (2016) provides tacit support for this suggestion by asserting that the central matter for resolution is the way in which people who have apportioned themselves an unreasonable slice of the resource pie should be addressed. Stiglitz (2011) is even clearer in his position that taxation policies favouring wealthy people are a large part of the reason for so much inequity in the US. Stiglitz (2011) is even clearer in his position that taxation policies favouring wealthy people are a large part of the reason for so much inequity in the US. Stiglitz (2011) contends that growing inequity is just one side of a coin. Shrinking opportunity is the other side. We will return to Stiglitz's views in the final chapter because they are not only monumentally profound in their scope but they are also eerily compatible with the PCT approach to deconstructing inequity and foretelling its long-term consequences.

If We Define Health Differently, We Might Study It Differently Too

When health is considered from the perspective of control, there seems to be sufficient justification, at least from our perspective, to define health *as* control. We can consider health at all levels of biological, psychological, and social functioning without having to demarcate arbitrary lines between physical and mental health, for example. A control view of the world, however, impacts not only on the way we define health, it has implications for the way in which we study health. Appreciating that, as researchers, we are also controllers, might help us reflect on the way in which we undertake research activity as well as the conclusions we report. An appreciation of the process of control will also demolish our current attitudes to causality that are reflected in our research programs with subsequent reverberating effects on the way in which we collect and analyse data. These themes will be explored further in the next two chapters.

References

American Psychiatric Association. (2013). *Diagnostic and statistical manual of mental disorders* (5th ed.). Washington, DC: American Psychiatric Association.

Anand, S. (2002). The concern for equity in health. *Journal of Epidemiology and Community Health, 56*(7), 485–487.

Beckfield, J., Bambra, C., Eikemo, T. A., Huijts, T., McNamara, C., & Wendt, C. (2015). An institutional theory of welfare state effects on the distribution of population health. *Social Theory & Health, 13*(3–4), 227–244. https://doi.org/10.1057/sth.2015.19.

Bezruchka, S. (2014). Inequality kills. In D. C. Johnston (Ed.), *Divided: The perils of our growing inequality* (pp. 190–198). New York: The New Press.

Bircher, J. (2005). Towards a dynamic definition of health and disease. *Medicine, Health Care and Philosophy, 8,* 335–341.

Blazquez-Fernandez, C., Cantarero-Prieto, D., & Pascual-Saez, M. (2018). Does rising income inequality reduce life expectancy? New evidence for 26 European countries (1995–2014). *Global Economic Review: Perspectives on East Asian Economies and Industries, 47*(4), 464–479. https://doi.org/10.1080/1226508X.2018.1526098.

Bracken, M. B. (2013). *Risk, chance, and causation.* New Haven, CT: Yale University Press.

Burns, H. (2014). What causes health? *Journal of the Royal College of Physicians of Edinburgh, 44,* 103–105.

Cannon, W. (1932). *The wisdom of the body.* New York: W.W. Norton.

Carey, T. A. (2013). Defining Australian Indigenous wellbeing: Do we *really* want the answers? Implications for policy and practice. *Psychotherapy and Politics International, 11*(3), 182–194.

Carey, T. A. (2016). Health is control. *Annals of Behavioural Science, 2*(1), 13.

Carey, T. A. (2017). *Patient-perspective care: A new paradigm for health systems and services.* London: Routledge.

Carey, T. A., Mansell, W., & Tai, S. J. (2014). A biopsychosocial model based on negative feedback and control. *Frontiers of Human Neuroscience, 8,* article 94. https://doi.org/10.3389/fnhum.2014.00094. http://journal.frontiersin.org/Journal/10.3389/fnhum.2014.00094/abstract.

Davies, K. J. A. (2016). *'Adaptive homeostasis', Molecular Aspects of Medicine* (pp. 1–7). Elsevier Ltd. https://doi.org/10.1016/j.mam.2016.04.007.

Engel, G. L. (1977). The need for a new medical model: A challenge for biomedicine. *Science, 196*(4286), 129–136.

Engel, G. L. (1980). The clinical application of the biopsychosocial model. *American Journal of Psychiatry, 137,* 535–544.

Fung, J. (2016). *The obesity code: Unlocking the secrets of weight loss.* London: Scribe Publications.

Galderisi, S., Heinz, A., Kastrup, M., Beezhold, J., & Sartorius, N. (2015). Toward a new definition of mental health. *World Psychiatry, 14*(2), 231–233.

Gilbert, N. (2016). *Never enough: Capitalism and the progressive spirit.* Oxford: Oxford University Press.

Haack, P., & Sieweke, J. (2018). The legitimacy of inequality: Integrating the perspectives of system justification and social judgment. *Journal of Management Studies, 55*(3), 486–516. https://doi.org/10.1111/joms.12323.

Hengartner, M. P., & Lehmann, S. N. (2017) Why psychiatric research must abandon traditional diagnostic classification and adopt a fully dimensional scope: Two solutions to a persistent problem. *Frontiers in Psychiatry.* Frontiers Media S.A., 8(June), p. 101. https://doi.org/10.3389/fpsyt.2017.00101.

Huber, M., Knottnerus, J. A., Green, L., van der Horst, H., Jadad, A. R., Kromhout, D., … Smid, H. (2011). How should we define health? *BMJ, 343,* d4163. https://doi.org/10.1136/bmj.d4163.

Huber, M., van Vliet, M., Giezenberg, M., Winkens, B., Heerkens, Y., Dagnelie, P. C., & Knottnerus, J. A. (2016). Towards a 'patient-centred' operationalisation of the new dynamic concept of health: A mixed methods study. *BMJ Open, 5,* e010091. https://doi.org/10.1136/bmjopen-2015-010091.

Jablensky, A. (2016). Psychiatric classifications: Validity and utility. *World Psychiatry, 15*(1), 26–31. https://doi.org/10.1002/wps.20284. Blackwell Publishing Ltd.

Koplan, J. P., Bond, T. C., Merson, M. H., Reddy, K. S., Rodriguez, M. H., Sewankambo, N. K., & Wasserheit, J. N. (2009). Towards a common definition of global health. *Lancet, 373,* 1993–1995.

Kragten, N., & Rozer, J. (2017). The income inequality hypothesis revisited: Assessing the hypothesis using four methodological approaches. *Social Indicators Research, 131,* 1015–1033.

Lancet Editorial. (2009, March 7). What is health? The ability to adapt. *The Lancet, 373,* p. 781.

Mackenbach, J. P. (2017). Persistence of social inequalities in modern welfare states: Explanation of a paradox. *Scandinavian Journal of Public Health, 45,* 113–120.

Marken, R. S., & Carey, T. A. (2015). *Controlling people: The paradoxical nature of being human.* Brisbane: Australian Academic Press.

Marks, D. F. (2018). *A general theory of behaviour.* London: Sage.

Marmot, M. (2006). Health in an unequal world: Social circumstances, biology and disease. *Clinical Medicine, 6*(6), 559–572.

Marmot, M. (2015). *The health gap: The challenge of an unequal world.* London: Bloomsbury.

McLaren, N. (1998). A critical review of the biopsychosocial model. *Australian and New Zealand Journal of Psychiatry, 32,* 86–92. https://doi.org/10.3109/00048679809062712.

Moynihan, R., & Cassels, A. (2005). *Selling Sickness: How the world's biggest pharmaceutical companies are turning us all into patients.* New York: Nation Books.

National Health Strategy Working Party. (1989). *A national Aboriginal health strategy 1989.* Canberra, Australia: Office of Aboriginal and Torres Strait Islander Health.

OECD. (2008). *Growing unequal? Income distribution and poverty in OECD countries.* Paris: OECD Publishing. Accessed 12 September 2020. https://www.oecd.org/els/soc/growingunequalincomedistributionandpovertyinoecdcountries.htm.

Powers, W. T. (1973). *Behavior: The control of perception.* Chicago: Aldine.

Powers, W. T. (1992). CT psychology and social organizations. In W. T. Powers (Ed.), *Living control systems II: Selected papers of William T. Powers* (pp. 91–127). Gravel Switch, KY: Control Systems Group.

Powers, W. T. (2005). *Behavior: The control of perception* (2nd ed.). New Canaan, CT: Benchmark.

Saini, V., Garcia-Armesto, S., Klemperer, D., Paris, V., Elshaug, A. G., Brownlee, S., ... Fisher, E. S. (2017). Drivers of poor medical care. *Lancet, Published online 8 January.* http://dx.doi.org/10.1016/S0140-6736(16)30947-3.

Saracci, R. (1997). The World Health Organisation needs to reconsider its definition of health. *BMJ, 314,* 1409–1410.

Saylor, C. (2004). The circle of health: A health definition model. *Journal of Holistic Nursing, 22*(2), 98–115.

Solar, O., & Irwin, A. (2010). *A conceptual framework for action on the social determinants of health.* Social Determinants of Health Discussion Paper 2 (Policy and Practice). Geneva: World Health Organization. Accessed 12 September 2020. https://www.who.int/sdhconference/resources/ConceptualframeworkforactiononSDH_eng.pdf.

Stiglitz, J. (2011). Of the 1%, by the 1%, for the 1%. *Vanity Fair*, March 31. Accessed 12 September 2020. https://www.vanityfair.com/news/2011/05/top-one-percent-201105.

Timimi, S. (2014). No more psychiatric labels: Why formal psychiatric diagnostic systems should be abolished. *International Journal of Clinical and Health Psychology, 14,* 208–215.

Vernon, D., Lowe, R., Thill, S., & Ziemke, T. (2015). Embodied cognition and circular causality: On the role of constitutive autonomy in the reciprocal coupling of perception and action. *Frontiers in Psychology, 6,* 1660.

Whitaker, R., & Cosgrove, L. (2015). *Psychiatry under the influence: Institutional corruption, social injury, and prescription for reform.* New York: Palgrave Macmillan.

Wilkinson, R., & Pickett, K. (2018). *The Inner level: How more equal societies reduce stress, restore sanity and improve everyone's well-being*. London: Penguin Random House.

WHO. (1946). *Constitution of the World Health Organization.* Accessed 12 September 2020. https://apps.who.int/gb/bd/PDF/bd47/EN/constitution-en.pdf?ua=1.

WHO. (2017). *Health is a fundamental human right.* Accessed 12 September 2020. https://www.who.int/mediacentre/news/statements/fundamental-human-right/en/.

CHAPTER 5

Research Through the Lens of Control: Reflecting on What We're Doing from a Different Vantage Point

Truth does not change because it is, or is not believed by a majority of the people. Giordano Bruno

As we pass the halfway mark of the book, it might be appropriate to take stock of where we have come from, and exactly what we are suggesting. During the years we've been writing about and teaching Perceptual Control Theory (PCT; Powers, 1973, 2005), we've noticed some typical responses from people when they first encounter organic, autonomous control as an object of investigation. Of course, everyone has been experiencing control for their whole life. Control, in fact, is why they have a life to experience. An unexpected rendezvous with control as a phenomenon of scientific enquiry, however, can be confronting. Engaging with the principles of PCT, along with the implications of those principles, can lead people to question implicit but fundamental assumptions about what it means to be human, the purpose of life, how we organise our affairs, how we structure and coordinate our communities, and the kind of society in which we want to live.

Common responses we've encountered include statements that control is too simple to explain all behaviour, but also, curiously, that it is too complex to account for simple behaviours. More generally, complexity is also used, on occasion, to explain how disadvantaged we are in the behavioural sciences compared with scientists in the physical sciences who,

T. A. Carey et al., *Deconstructing Health Inequity*,
https://doi.org/10.1007/978-3-030-68053-4_5

apparently, study much more straightforward phenomena. The relevance of this point to the phenomenon of control is that we think any object or event seems complex, perhaps even magical, before it is understood accurately and precisely. As Arthur C. Clarke famously asserted, "Any sufficiently advanced technology is indistinguishable from magic" (Clarke, 1973). When we don't understand how something works, it can appear baffling or even mystical. We have also been advised that people are not machines and that more advanced models have already superseded negative feedback control. All of these remarks are entirely understandable efforts to nullify the disturbance that the phenomenon of control poses, when one gets some hints about the type of phenomenon it is and begins to appreciate the ramifications it forebodes.

We Are All Controllers All the Time

Control is us, from before those first two cells do their human creating tango until that last breath is released into the world. We are all controllers. All the time.

Taking the leap, from where we are now, to understanding people as controllers, has implications that reach far beyond simply reconfiguring the way we conceptualise and define health. If people are controllers, then the principles of control apply just as much to researchers, politicians, health professionals, and policymakers, as they do to people who participate in researchers' programs of enquiry, or who seek the assistance of health professionals. In terms of understanding and eradicating health inequity, current efforts have been informed by attitudes, beliefs, and strategies that are, in many ways, inconsistent with our design as organic, autonomous control systems. In particular, a number of existing conditions and circumstances could be considered to have combined in such a way to have produced a perfect storm of blind alleys, dead ends, misleading conclusions, unfulfilled promises, and contradictions. We would especially identify: a failure to recognise the implicit goals of researchers; the ubiquity of linear models of causality; an almost complete reliance on statistical significance as a benchmark for scientific importance; and the preponderance of aggregated data, as keys to the current situation. The amalgam of all these factors has meant that the answers to how the physical, psychological, and social functioning of individuals might be improved on a widespread, equitable, and sustainable scale are still nowhere to be seen. Consequently, the collaborative efforts of researchers, policymakers, health professionals, and other people of influence to discover, organise, and mobilise the factors that will enable the cohesive harmonisation of communities is also still beyond the horizon.

Researchers as Controllers

As researchers, clinicians, and educators, we are aware of our own controlling natures. The reason we have spent time explaining how we came to write this book, and some of our adventures during that undertaking, is so that you might gain some appreciation of *our* goals and motivations. We have found it enormously beneficial, both in our professional and personal lives, to be clear, not only about the goals that are important to us, but also the way these goals influence other goals, as well as where we focus our attention. Some goals, for example, change the settings of less complex goals as their means of keeping the aspect of the world that is relevant to them in its preferred state. The goal that keeps your car in a certain position on the road, does so by varying the goals for the way in which the steering wheel is manoeuvred, and this is achieved by those goals altering the goals for various muscle tensions in your arms and hands and shoulders. Similarly, in our clinical work we achieve goals for helping people resolve psychological distress, by varying goals for the questions we ask, what we ask questions about, the timing and pacing of the questions, and so on. Higher-order goals such as "leaving the world in a better state than I found it", might be achieved by setting goals related to conducting programs of research, which will involve goals about formulating important research questions, selecting methodologies, and collecting and analysing data.

At any point in time, the control systems that have the greatest separation between their goal standard, and the ceaselessly streaming report they receive from the world, are the ones that will command your attention. Things that are not right, are very difficult to genuinely ignore for any length of time. And "not right", for entities that control, *always* means a situation that needs rectifying in terms of matching the world report with the goal standard.

As we have explained, achieving greater precision and accuracy in the behavioural sciences, is a goal that informs many of *our* decisions in the work that we do. It was the increasing disturbance to that goal, as we became better and better acquainted with the health inequity literature, that generated goals for preparing book proposals, arranging regular meetings, composing drafts of chapters, and so on. The words you are now reading, came to be selected and arranged the way they are through our controlling, which involved a cascading process of goal adjustment and achievement. Ultimately, the word sequencing process also involved the controlling of editors, publishers, and partners and friends who all contemplated to differing degrees, these words, or variations of them.

We mentioned earlier, particularly in Chapter 2, the different methodological decisions that researchers make, and the influence those decisions have on the way in which results are eventually reported. All of these deliberations are part of the researchers' controlling to make their worlds be right. The results you encounter, in the form you encounter them, provide evidence of the goals and controlling efforts of those particular researchers. In Chapter 2, we referred to McIntyre's (2019, p. 297) suggestion that "some researchers will discover results that are squarely in line with liberal political beliefs, while others will produce conservative results that are directly opposed to them". McIntyre (2019) is, unwittingly, referring to control processes. Such is the inescapable ubiquity of control. We will consider the controlling of two researchers with regard to one particular study in some detail in Chapter 7.

Examples of Researchers' Controlling

In Chapter 2, we provided what we consider a clear example of how the same control process can lead to different outcomes, depending on the different preferences, standards, and proclivities of different researchers. That instance concerned the relationship between homicide and income inequity. In one reporting of the apparent homicide-income inequity association, Wilkinson and Pickett (2010) describe a statistically significant relationship (we have more to say about statistical significance in Chapter 6) between homicide and income inequity. They provide Fig. 10.2 to illustrate the relationship (Wilkinson & Pickett, 2010). Gilbert (2016), however, sees the situation differently. From Gilbert's (2016) perspective, the data point provided by the United States (US) in this figure, is so extreme, that omitting it as an outlier would be well-justified. Saunders (2010, p. 29, Fig. 6), in fact, provides a boxplot test to verify how extreme the US is as an outlier. If the US was not included, the relationship between homicide and income inequity would no longer be statistically significant. So, should the US be included in the calculations and subsequent reporting, or not? Justification can be, and in fact was, provided for either decision based entirely on the controlling of the justifiers, the goal states being maintained.

When a control perspective is adopted, new options for assessing statements and claims emerge. Not only can the accuracy and precision of the various pronouncements be appraised, but the controlling, in terms of the goals being tended, can also be pondered. Wilkinson and Pickett (2018), for example, report that "the proportion of the labour force employed in what has been called 'guard' labour (such as security staff, police and prison officers) increases as income differences get larger" (p. 228). Perhaps the first thing to notice with this assertion is that it is reporting a *correlation* between income differences and the proportion of the labour force employed as guard labour. Although the particular word sequence that Wilkinson and Pickett (2018) used to express the relationship is strongly suggestive of causality, not even an inkling of causality is appropriate in this situation. A correlation makes no statement about causality (a point we will expand on below). So, the words could just as accurately have been expressed in the form "income differences get larger as guard labour increases", but perhaps arranging the words in this way would not have conveyed the message that Wilkinson and Pickett (2018) favoured.

When the references provided by Wilkinson and Pickett (2018) for this relationship are consulted, further evidence emerges of the way in which different outcomes can arise from the same control process, according to the different goal states of different researchers. In two papers discussing the relationship between guard labour and income differences, Jayadev and Bowles (2006) and Bowles and Jayadev (2007) remind readers that "None of the statistical associations we have presented are properly identified causal relationships" (Bowles & Jayadev, 2007, pp. 4–5; Jayadev & Bowles, 2006, p. 343). Inspecting the figure that illustrates the rise in guard labour from 1890 to 2002 in the US (Bowles & Jayadev, 2007, p. 3, Fig. 1) also reveals a conundrum in reconciling its association with income inequity. The figure shows a constant increase in guard labour from 1890 to 2002, yet it is well established that income inequity has had a much more variable journey across that time span. According to Bowles and Jayadev (2007, p. 5), "the long term growth in guard labor in the United States cannot be explained by inequality trends, or at least not in any simple way, because income inequality fell over most of the last century before rising during the past three decades". And so, we have two statements about the same research from the same set of data:

> *the proportion of the labour force employed in what has been called 'guard' labour (such as security staff, police and prison officers) increases as income differences get larger* (Wilkinson & Pickett, 2018, p. 228);

and

> *the long term growth in guard labor in the United States cannot be explained by inequality trends* (Bowles & Jayadev, 2007, p. 5).

Two *different* word sequences by two *different* sets of authors conveying two *different* impressions about the *same* data. We think the juxtaposition of these statements is potent evidence of the phenomenon of control, in which both sets of researchers acted to keep their worlds in the states that are right for them.

Saunders (2010, p. 21), in his critique of Wilkinson and Pickett's (2010) book *The Spirit Level*, provides further examples of the way in which different results can be achieved even when similar processes are followed. For instance, starting with the same population of 50 countries from which Wilkinson and Pickett (2010) derived their final sample of 23 countries, Saunders (2010), by using the same decision-making process with slightly different criteria (such as an exclusionary population cut-off of 1 million rather than less than 3 million), arrives at a final sample of 44 countries. Later, by mimicking Wilkinson and Pickett's (2010) procedural logic but with different variables, Saunders (2010, p. 107) is able to justify a conclusion that "as countries become more equal, life gets more miserable". This conclusion is diametrically opposed to that which is offered by Wilkinson and Pickett (2010).

The research process is one way in which some people, namely researchers, control a variety of things that are important to them. Perceptions don't just shape reality (Stiglitz, 2012). Perceptions are the entirety of our reality and, as the title of Powers's (1973, 2005) book suggests, our behaviour is a process of controlling those perceptions in terms of the goals, plans, expectations, proclivities, standards, preferences, hopes and dreams, tendencies, propensities, beliefs, and other specifications by which we are defined. "Research behaviour" is just one of the means we use to keep our worlds in the states they must be in.

We recently happened upon a quote that seemed provocatively relevant:

It doesn't matter how many resources you have …
If you don't know how to use them, it will never be enough.[1]

We would apply this to the health inequity area by offering that:

It doesn't matter how many studies you conduct …
If you're using the wrong model, it will never be enough.

It Doesn't Matter How Closely We Scrutinise Inequity

Since we are controllers, problems will occur whenever our controlling is obstructed, impeded, or otherwise impaired. Control systems are very good, ordinarily, at opposing disturbances to maintain equilibrium, balance, and alignment between private standards and their idiosyncratic experiencing of the world. That is, in fact, what control is. The reason that control is necessary, is because the world is jam-packed with unpredictably varying states and conditions. Something that doesn't vary, doesn't need to be controlled. Our perceptions, however, composed of those different aspects of our cacophonous surroundings that buffet and caress our senses, constantly vary. Or at least they would, if we were not so good at controlling them.

There are many ways in fact, in which control efforts can be scuppered. A daily menu of half a small bowl of rice will not be able to sustain adequate controlling for very long. Extended periods without sleep, living in unsafe environments, prolonged exposure to pathogens and toxins, and being unable to protect one's body temperature and skin exposure against the vagaries of the daily weather conditions, will all similarly compromise control.

Problems are only problems because they interfere with control. As we proposed at the end of Chapter Three, inequity and unfairness will be problems solely to the extent that they impede or obstruct control. Inequity per se is not a problem. Unfairness per se is not a problem. Compromised control *is* the problem. Our suggestion, then, is not that

[1] https://www.yourquote.in/justice-osei-1sw2/quotes/it-doesnt-matter-how-many-resources-you-have-you-dont-know-midoh.

we should abandon research efforts that explore matters of inequity. Rather, we are offering that research efforts might coalesce into a cohesive and powerfully persuasive message, if the object of enquiry was more nuanced and finessed than simply health inequity, social inequity, or any of the other variants on this theme that we have encountered. Inequity enquiries need to focus on the ways in which control can be compromised through the organisation of inequitable conditions and circumstances. Control is what we do. Therefore, to discover how we can help individuals and the communities they create, do what they do, and do it as well as they would like, control must be fundamental to our explorations and investigations.

It Doesn't Matter How Many Linear Causal Pathways We Construct

So endemic is the linear model of causality that we would not be surprised if most researchers don't even know that they subscribe to it. Some are aware of this, of course, and embrace it with gusto. As we will demonstrate below, if the frequency with which something is mentioned is any indication of its priority, then the conclusion must be that linear causality is highly esteemed in the health inequity literature. Unfortunately, with scientific activity, it is evidence, rather than the number of people who agree, that must be the standard (McIntyre, 2019). Yet, in the inequity arena, researchers en masse appear committed to understanding causality as a linear line from A to B. A is usually, but not always, income inequity, and B is frequently, though not exclusively, some aspect of health or social problems.

We take no issue with efforts to understand the processes by which something arises. We also applaud attempts to elucidate the manifestation of a particular problem or situation. We do think, however, that it is prudent to scrutinise *all* aspects of the research process, including the model upon which research assumptions are based. In fact, using the results of experiments to modify and improve existing theories and models is an essential aspect of the complete scientific process (McIntyre, 2019). Unfortunately, this part of the process is often neglected in the behavioural sciences. An attitude of examining underlying theories and models, however, is very much a part of the meta-methods we have previously mentioned. The fundamental problem with a non-critical examination of the linear model applied to living things is that, in the context of entities that live, it is the wrong model.

The lavishly indiscriminate adoption of the linear model is, of course, much more widespread than the inequity field. Yin (2013), in fact, states that the linear causation paradigm is the dominant paradigm with regard to the study of behaviour in fields such as psychology and neuroscience. Yet, despite its pervasive influence, “linear causation does not apply to any control system with negative feedback” (Yin, 2013, p. 319). “Any control system with negative feedback” includes every living thing. Our focus in this book is the health inequity domain. It is important to acknowledge, however, the unquestioned and almost complete universality of the linear model, as well as the extent of its inappropriateness for the study of the process of living. Information about the inadequacy of the linear model has been available to us for a long time:

> *A number of psychological theories popular in the first half of this century attempt to explain behaviour in terms of simple stimulus-response (S-R) reflexes that are chained together in various ways. Unfortunately, these theories were popular in the curriculum of psychology courses and became part of many students’ understanding of reflexes. Studies by Sherrington and subsequently by other physiologists showed that even the simplest reflexes in the spinal cord provide little support for these theories. Sensory receptors that supply the spinal cord with input act as filters in that they are selective about the features of the stimuli to which they respond. The reflexes that a stimulus elicits are not related in a one-to-one fashion to either the duration or the intensity of the stimulation.* (Kolb & Wishaw, 1990, p. 165)

If the linear model cannot even adequately explain simple stimulus-response reflexes, what hope can it possibly have of explaining the vast array of highly complex behaviours exhibited by living things?

It’s Loops Not Lines When It Comes to Causality

Linear causality is an enduring theme throughout the inequity literature. It is, in fact, difficult to read a book or a journal article about inequity without encountering some statement of, or reference to, a linearly causal process. But it doesn’t matter how earnestly we study linear causality in relation to inequity. The linear model will never help us understand, accurately and precisely, the impact of inequity on social living, because social living is control.

It is true that if you take a small enough segment of a circle, it will appear to be a straight line. Understanding the intricacies and properties of that minuscule non-curved element, however, will, ultimately, be of very little value unless it is placed back within the whole unit, and its contribution to the circularity of which it is an essential component, is acknowledged. Our contention is that the efforts in the inequity field have been scrutinising various straight-line aspects of inequity without ever placing those fragments back into the nonlinear process from which they were extracted.

The General State of the Literature with Regard to Causality

At the risk of being accused of "cherry picking", we felt some selected examples could provide a sense of the general tone of the inequity literature as it appeared to us. Clouston, Rubin, Phelan, and Link (2016) mention risk factors that might be "lying between SES [socioeconomic status] and disease in a causal chain" (p. 1633). Curran and Mahutga (2018) refer to a "causal link" (p. 537) between inequity and health as well as the "causal path from inequality to health" (p. 540). Moreover, they suggest that theories which link income inequity and poor health at a population level "provide compelling causal mechanisms" (p. 548). In Chapter 2, we referred to Pickett and Wilkinson's (2015) causal review performed within an epidemiological causal framework which, they report, enabled them to infer the "likelihood of a causal relationship between income inequality and health" (p. 316). They refer to Hill's (1965) causal criteria and suggest that, in their review, the four most important criteria of the original nine that Hill presented, were satisfied. Their assertion is that the body of evidence strongly indicates a causal connection between income inequity and health (Pickett & Wilkinson, 2015). Rothstein and Uslaner (2005), in a paper discussing the importance of social trust, "argue that inequality stands at the beginning of the causal chain" and, in the next paragraph, "Equality and honesty in government stand at the beginning of our causal chain" (p. 44). Diderichsen (2010, p. 3) in the Foreword to Solar and Irwin (2010) refers to "long causal chains". Throughout their comprehensive volume titled *A conceptual framework for action on the social determinants of health*, published by the World Health Organization (WHO), Solar and Irwin (2010) make reference to: "the causal priority" (p. 6); "causal pathways" (pp. 9, 30) and "causal pathway" (p. 47); "causal hierarchies" (pp. 9, 30); "causal linkages" (p. 12) and "causal links" (p. 18); the "causal effect of socioeconomic status on health" (p. 17) which they describe as being "likely to be mainly indirect" (p. 17); "the causal processes that underlie health inequities" (p. 20); "causal factors" (pp. 23, 40) and "a causal factor" (p. 38); "causal and temporal ordering" (p. 29); a "causal chain" (pp. 31, 47); the social determinants of health being "causally antecedent" to other determinants; a "causal relationship" (p. 37) and "causal relationships" (p. 55); "the causal complex" (p. 38); "causal areas" (p. 39); and "the causal priority" (pp. 45, 64). Stafford, Bartley, Mitchell, and Marmot (2001) refer to a "causal pathway between individual social position and health" (p. 118). Barr, Bambra, and Smith (2016) recommend going beyond the dominant paradigm of causality to consider an "alternative 'realist' conception of causality" (p. 253). The realist depiction they offer requires an understanding not only of any hypothesised causal mechanism responsible for the connection between cause and effect, but also the contextual factors upon which the connection supposedly relies. While we unconditionally support a consideration of context, the portrayal of causality recommended by Barr et al. (2016) still preserves the linear march from a cause to an effect. Wilkinson and Pickett (2018) are others who freely discuss causality in various ways such as: "a causal role" (p. xx); "causal mechanisms" (p. xx); "causal processes" (pp. xxiii, 17, 201); "multi-causal" (p. 9); and "causal pathways" (p. 154). Wilkinson and Pickett (2010) describe the relationship between inequity and different health outcomes as "strong" and go on to explain their justification for the "belief that this is a causal relationship" (p. 99).

Some People Seem to Know Something Is Amiss

We do not back away at all from our claim that the overwhelming taste left in one's mouth after feasting on the health inequity literature, is one of linear causality. There are, however, much to our delight, hints every now and then, like tasty little morsels, of a growing awareness that the notion of linearity is, somehow, not quite right. Even Wilkinson and Pickett (2017), for example, despite their predilection for all things linearly causal, admit that there is little understanding of the processes that make income inequity the problem it seems to be. To us, this lack of understanding makes perfect sense given the glaring absence of any functional description or model regarding the way in which the causality that is discussed, works. When descriptions remain only at the word level, there is a much greater latitude of possibilities for what can be proposed than there is when ideas are submitted to the much more exacting standard of building a functional model that demonstrates how the ideas actually work. Even testing assumptions through statistical procedures does not come close to the results that can be achieved through functional models.

When referring to models, some authorities contend that "the causal arrows are likely to run in both directions" (Wilkinson & Pickett, 2010, p. 55), and also that, "In many of my examples, one could reverse the arrow of the effects of social capital, and tell a story where the arrow runs to social capital instead of from social capital" (Putnam, 2001, p. 14). Putnam (2001), however, also admits that, with regard to social capital, "There is no way to be entirely sure in which direction causality runs" (p. 11). Schneider (2019) refers to "reversed causality" (p. 424), and Wilkinson and Pickett (2018) mention situations where "it becomes difficult to understand causal pathways at all" (p. 154). With regard to the specific relationship between participation in the arts and national income differences, for example, Wilkinson and Pickett (2018, p. 201) offer that, "There are several possible causal processes that might account for this finding". Rothstein and Uslaner (2005, p. 57) refer to "causal cycles" within which different countries are proposed to operate.

Encouragingly, at times references are made to something called "feedback". When we encountered these references, however, the feedback term was encased in quotation marks. Moreover, there appeared to be little appreciation of the type of feedback that was important, or its significance as a functional, physical mechanism. Rothstein and Uslaner (2005), for example, seem almost apologetic when they "admit there are "feedback mechanisms"" (p. 46). We mentioned above that Rothstein and Uslaner (2005, p. 44) nominate the variables that are at the beginning of their causal chain, yet they also contend that "reinforcing effects of inequality and honesty on trust and social policy - and the "feedback" to greater trust and less inequality - lead to a positive equilibrium for societies". Solar and Irwin (2010) also refer to feedback, however, not only do they surround the term with quotation marks they also include a space to make two words out of one. Nevertheless, Solar and Irwin (2010) seem to admit that something other than linear causality might be occurring when they suggest that "Illness can "feed back" on a given individual's social position, e.g. by compromising employment opportunities and reducing income; certain epidemic diseases can similarly "feed back" to affect the functioning of social, economic and political institutions" (p. 5).

Every Now and then an Exciting Glimmer of Circular Causality Appears

It is possible to find statements that indicate recognition, if only conceptually, of a circularity of causality that might be present. At times, Solar and Irwin (2010) go beyond simply mentioning "feed back". They suggest, for example, that "the causal linkages between health and agency are not uni-directional" (p. 12). Not only are they not uni-directional, but Solar and Irwin (2010) clarify that "health enables agency, but greater agency and freedom also yield better health" (p. 12). To perhaps illustrate the tightness of the grip maintained by the current paradigm of linear causality and controlled behavioural output, however, Solar and Irwin (2010) refer to this blurring of linear cause and effect as the "mutually reinforcing nature" (p. 12) of the relationship. Even though Garnham (2015) refers to pathways through which the availability of capital and various actions can influence health, she also states that "aspects of a place are both shaped by and provide shape to strategies of action" (p. 317).

From information outside the health inequity field, Vernon, Lowe, Thill, and Ziemke (2015, para. 1) are unambiguous and direct with their reference to circular causality when they insist that the "reciprocal coupling of perception and action in cognitive agents has been firmly established: perceptions guide action but so too do actions influence what is perceived". Despite their unequivocal position regarding circular causality, there is evidence that failing to include a functional model in their cogitations might have limited the scope of their work. For example, they conclude that "It remains as a significant research challenge to uncover the specific mechanisms by which circular causality and allostasis arise in natural agents and how—and to what degree—they might be replicated in artificial systems" (Vernon et al., 2015, "Conclusion", para. 1). They seem to be unaware of the phenomenon of control established through negative feedback, and that this natural phenomenon is mimicked in devices such as cruise control systems in motor vehicles, and temperature regulation systems in buildings.

Within the health inequity territory, a particularly clear description of an alternative formulation to linear conceptualisations is provided by

Saunders (2010). Saunders (2010) also provides a counter to the strategy of demarcating an arbitrary starting point in an imagined linear progression. Saunders (2010) invokes an evolutionary process when he explains that "Sweden and Japan, for example, have the income distributions they have because of the kinds of societies they are. They are not cohesive societies because their incomes are equally distributed; their incomes are equally distributed because they evolved as remarkably cohesive societies" (p. 8).

But with the Wrong Model We're Still Asking the Wrong Questions

Despite occasional but encouraging counterpoints to the dominant narrative of linear causality, the stranglehold this model has on our thinking should not be underestimated. Raphael and Bryant (2015), for example, when considering the effects of public policies associated with welfare states, suggest that we should be asking how "social determinants and their distribution (associated with varying welfare state types) mediate the vulnerabilities of those occupying specific social locations)" (p. 251). The idea of particular variables *mediating* relationships and processes between other variables is another commonly expressed notion throughout the inequity literature. This is a further concept that is as incorrectly incomplete as linear causality. We are not mediating creatures. We are controllers. Seeking to answer questions relating to illusory mediating processes will not move us closer to eradicating those factors that persistently and pervasively mar people's ability to control. The novelist Kurt Vonnegut expresses this sentiment eloquently when he says:

> *That is the first thing I know for sure: (1.) If the questions don't make sense, neither will the answers.*[2]

But Wait! There's More …

The name of the game is control. Once an attitude of control informs the scrutiny of a particular undertaking there is, quite literally, no corner into which the light won't shine. We have introduced some of the implications of an inspection of research activity from the perspective of control.

[2] https://www.goodreads.com/quotes/930495-that-is-the-first-thing-i-know-for-sure-1.

In particular, it is important to recognise researchers as controllers and also to be prepared for the way in which an understanding of control clarifies what the important topics to investigate might be. Crucially, the phenomenon of control has unforgiving messages for the way we understand and address causality. We explore this theme further in the next chapter and also suggest some ways in which we could start to make things matter with the winds of control at our back.

References

Barr, B., Bambra, C., & Smith, K. E. (2016). For the good of the cause: Generating evidence to inform social policies that reduce health inequalities. In K. E. Smith, S. Hill, & C. Bambra (Eds.), *Health inequalities: Critical perspectives* (pp. 252–264). Oxford: Oxford University Press.

Bowles, S., & Jayadev, A. (2007). Garrison America. *Economists' Voice, 4*(2), 1–7.

Clarke, A. C. (1973). *Profiles of the future: An inquiry into the limits of the possible* (Rev. ed.). New York: Harper & Row. ISBN 978-0-33023619-5.

Clouston, S. A. P., Rubin, M. S., Phelan, J. C., & Link, B. G. (2016). A social history of disease: Contextualizing the rise and fall of social inequalities in cause-specific mortality. *Demography, 53,* 1631–1656. https://doi.org/10.1007/s13524-106-0495-5.

Curran, M., & Mahutga, M. C. (2018). Income inequality and population health: A global gradient? *Journal of Health and Social Behavior, 59*(4), 536–553.

Diderichsen, F. (2010). Foreword. In O. Solar & A. Irwin (Eds.), *A conceptual framework for action on the social determinants of health.* Social Determinants of Health Discussion Paper 2 (Policy and Practice) (p. 3). Geneva: World Health Organization. Accessed 12 September 2020. https://www.who.int/sdhconference/resources/ConceptualframeworkforactiononSDH_eng.pdf.

Garnham, L. M. (2015). Understanding the impacts of industrial change and area-based deprivation on health inequalities, using Swidler's concepts of cultured capacities and strategies of action. *Social Theory & Health, 13*(3–4), 308–339.

Gilbert, N. (2016). *Never enough: Capitalism and the progressive spirit*. Oxford: Oxford University Press.

Hill, A. B. (1965). The environment and disease: Association or causation? *Proceedings of the Royal Society of Medicine, 58*(5), 295–300.

Jayadev, A., & Bowles, S. (2006). Guard labor. *Journal of Development Economics, 79*(2), 328–348.

Kolb, B., & Wishaw, I. Q. (1990). *Fundamentals of human neuropsychology*. New York: W. H. Freeman and Company.

McIntyre, L. (2019). *The scientific attitude: Defending science from denial, fraud, and pseudoscience*. Cambridge, MA: The MIT Press.

Pickett, K. E., & Wilkinson, R. G. (2015). Income inequality and health: A causal review. *Social Science and Medicine, 128,* 316–326.

Powers, W. T. (1973). *Behavior: The control of perception*. Chicago: Aldine.

Powers, W. T. (2005). *Behavior: The control of perception* (2nd ed.). New Canaan, CT: Benchmark.

Putnam, R. (2001). Social capital: Measurement and consequences. *Canadian Journal of Policy Research*. Accessed 12 September 2020. http://www.sietmanagement.fr/wp-content/uploads/2016/04/Putnam_SocialCapital.pdf.

Raphael, D., & Bryant, T. (2015). Power, intersectionality and the life-course: Identifying the political and economic structures of welfare states that support or threaten health. *Social Theory & Health, 13*(3–4), 245–266. https://doi.org/10.1057/sth.2015.18.

Rothstein, B., & Uslaner, E. M. (2005). All for all: Equality, corruption, and social trust. *World Politics, 58*(1), 41–72.

Saunders, P. (2010). *Beware false prophets: Equality, the good society, and the Spirit Level*. London: Policy Exchange. Accessed 30 September 2020. https://www.policyexchange.org.uk/wp-content/uploads/2016/09/beware-false-prophets-jul-10.pdf.

Schneider, S. M. (2019). Why income inequality is dissatisfying—Perceptions of social status and the inequality-satisfaction link in Europe. *European Sociological Review, 35*(3), 409–430. https://doi.org/10.1093/esr/jcz003.

Solar, O., & Irwin, A. (2010). *A conceptual framework for action on the social determinants of health*. Social Determinants of Health Discussion Paper 2 (Policy and Practice). Geneva: World Health Organization. Accessed 12 September 2020. https://www.who.int/sdhconference/resources/ConceptualframeworkforactiononSDH_eng.pdf.

Stafford, M., Bartley, M., Mitchell, R., & Marmot, M. (2001). Characteristics of individuals and characteristics of areas: Investigating their influence on health in the Whitehall II study. *Health & Place, 7,* 117–129.

Stiglitz, J. E. (2012). *The price of inequality: How today's divided society endangers our future*. New York: W. W. Norton & Company.

Vernon, D., Lowe, R., Thill, S., & Ziemke, T. (2015). Embodied cognition and circular causality: On the role of constitutive autonomy in the reciprocal coupling of perception and action. *Frontiers in Psychology, 6,* 1660.

Wilkinson, R., & Pickett, K. (2010). *The spirit level: Why equality is better for everyone*. London: Penguin Books.

Wilkinson, R. G., & Pickett, K. E. (2017). The enemy between us: The psychological and social costs of inequality. *European Journal of Social Psychology, 47,* 11–24.

Wilkinson, R., & Pickett, K. (2018). *The Inner level: How more equal societies reduce stress, restore sanity and improve everyone's well-being*. London: Penguin Random House.

Yin, H. H. (2013). Restoring purpose in behavior. In G. Baldassarre & M. Mirolli (Eds.), *Computational and robotic models of the hierarchical organization of behaivor* (pp. 319–347). London: Springer.

CHAPTER 6

Supercharging Our Research Efforts: A Matter of Control

In questions of science, the authority of a thousand is not worth the humble reasoning of a single individual. Galileo Galilei

We suggested in the last chapter that understanding our controlling natures might have important and useful implications for the way in which we conduct research. These implications will include unambiguous lessons for the issues we research and the research questions we develop and seek to answer. The ways in which we analyse data and the models we construct are other aspects of the research process that would be advanced by an understanding of control. An appreciation of control and how it occurs permits a realigning of attitudes and beliefs so that the research we do might actually start to matter for the global community we serve.

It Doesn't Matter How Complex Our Statistical Analyses Are

If what is being studied in the inequity area, in terms of a model of linear causality, is incorrect, then it perhaps makes some sense that the way in which research is being conducted might also be incorrect. We would suggest that an almost complete reliance on statistical analyses and models to build our understanding of inequity and its impact is not so much

T. A. Carey et al., *Deconstructing Health Inequity*,
https://doi.org/10.1007/978-3-030-68053-4_6

incorrect as it is incomplete. This incompleteness will be showcased in the next chapter in terms of one specific study.

Currently, we are demanding much more of statistical methods than they can reasonably deliver. And because there is a colossal mismatch between the nature of what we are studying and the methods we are using to study it, we have had to make certain adjustments such as studying groups of individuals and relying on aggregated data. Once again, Yin's (2013, p. 321) insights are instructive:

> *The statistically average animal appears to show the stimulus-response correlation that satisfies the experimenter, even if the individual animal does not. Whereas neuroscience has focused on the "partial animal," so that whatever is left can "behave" according to the experimenter's* a priori *assumptions about what behavior should be, psychology studies the "average animal", or the "Gaussian animal," a creature not found in the woods.*

We'll Never Spin Correlations into Causation

A great deal of the research conducted in the health inequity field considers the way in which some variables change in relation to other variables. Regression models are also quite common in which statistical models are constructed that predict, with varying levels of accuracy, the value of one variable from the value of another variable or combinations of two or more variables. Both correlation, and the regression models that are typically used in this area, make straightforward assumptions about the linear relationship between the variables under consideration. We are aware that regression models can also be nonlinear, although, the use of nonlinear regression models in the behavioural sciences is very rare (Malkina-Pykh & Pykh, 2019). Linear regression, on the other hand, is widely used. Both correlation and regression, however, are techniques of association rather than causation (Pearl, 2009).

Wilkinson and Pickett (2018, p. xviii) contend that "the evidence is now such that these correlations between income inequality and both health and social problems must be regarded as causal". Unfortunately, causality doesn't work that way. Gilbert (2016, p. 71) reminds us that "every research student knows that correlations do not confirm causality, even if there are many leaning in the same direction". It is simply not the case that:

$$correlation + correlation + \ldots + correlation = causation$$

or, to put it another way

$$n(correlation) = causation \text{ (where n > 1)}$$

Much more serious, however, than the link between correlation and causation is the way in which correlations can behave when a control system is the object of investigation. In Experiments 1–5 in Chapter 3, for example, extraordinarily high correlations were recorded between Tim's (first author) actions and an unseen, unknown, and unpredictable computer-generated movement pattern. Despite the high correlations, it would be silly to suggest that one of these variables caused the changes in the other. Silly, and yet, in a way, contextually correct. Kennaway (1998) has studied how correlations between variables behave with control systems. The results can be baffling and even disconcerting. Such is the profound importance of understanding how control systems work. If control systems are present, in fact, "causal analysis from correlational data is not possible" (Kennaway, 1998, p. 12). Moreover, "It is a characteristic of control systems in general, that the outputs by which they control their perceptions have very low correlations with those perceptions, although each continuously causes the other" (Kennaway, 1998, p. 12). It is also important to be aware that, whenever dynamical systems are being studied, such as the kind of systems described by the equations of control theory, "No causal analysis based on correlational data is capable of yielding a correct description" (Kennaway, 1998, p. 11). Finally, when relationships between variables are investigated using standard techniques such as analysis of variance, not only does correlation not imply causality but it cannot be assumed "that either variable has any causal influence on the other" (Kennaway, 1998, p. 3).

Statistics Are Good but They Are Not That Good

Statistical analysis is of fundamental importance in the behavioural sciences. It is critical, however, to be clear about what statistical analyses can and cannot do. Scambler and Scambler (2015) confess that statistical associations can only hint at causal mechanisms. Schneider (2019) recommends that to explore fundamental questions about the mechanisms linking income inequity and life satisfaction, we need more nuanced statistical analyses. Pearl (2009) provides detailed guidance of the way in which causal inference can be conducted in statistics. Yet, despite the power and usefulness of these methods, as we stated above, they are not relevant to, and, in fact, can be misleading in, studies in which control systems are present (Kennaway, 1998).

We would offer that it doesn't matter how intricate and complex our statistical analyses become, they will never produce the answers we seek in terms of how organisms function. We need to use statistical analysis to achieve the purpose for which it was designed. Then, we need to gain an understanding of the way in which control systems function, and adopt methods that are suited to, and appropriate for, understanding that functioning with accuracy and precision.

The Scientific Insignificance of Statistical Significance

Given the almost total reliance on the statistical analysis of data for the production of research findings, it is unsurprising that statistical significance is the most common standard for judging the value or importance of a result. Readers of the inequity literature who are not well versed in empirical work might not always realise that, almost without exception, when "significance" or "significant" is referred to in the literature, this is, in the first instance at least, momentous only in a statistical sense. Significant, in this context, does not necessarily equate with important or meaningful. Wilkinson and Pickett (2010, p. 272), for example, assert that "Our results are, of course, sometimes sensitive to exclusions simply because we are looking at a limited number of countries, but the fact that so many relationships with inequality are statistically significant, despite the limits to the data, is an indication of how powerful the underlying relationships actually are". Wilkinson and Pickett (2018, p. 205) report that they "used data from Child Rights International Network and found a statistically significant relationship between inequality and a lower age of criminal responsibility". Baek and Kim (2018, p. 192) describe the correlation between GDP per capita and life expectancy as demonstrating "very strong statistical significance". Pickett and Wilkinson (2015, p. 320) state that "A very large number of studies demonstrate statistically significant linear relationships between income inequality and health". Schneider (2019, p. 414) advises that "Only a few studies do not find a statistically significant association between income inequality and well-being in Europe".

Once again, we readily acknowledge that the inequity arena is not the only stadium where statistical significance has been assigned the privileged status of the equivalent of a home run. We would suggest that the points we raise apply generally. Our focus in this book, however, is inequity. Since "statistical significance" has been adopted as the signal for what should and should not be attended to, with regard to noteworthy findings about inequity and its impact, it is important to be very clear about just exactly what statistical significance tells us.

Bracken (2013, p. 273) suggests that "Compared to other sciences, the 1 in 20 criteria for an observation being unlikely due to chance, thereby being considered 'statistically significant' and so worthy of special attention because it may be causal, is quite liberal". In Chapter 3, we also included some cautions offered by Powers (1990) regarding the limitations of statistical generalisations. Coe (2002) reminds us that statistical significance depends only on the size of the effect and the size of the sample. Rosnow and Rosenthal (2013, p. 220) depict the relationship as:

$$\textit{Significance test} = \textit{Size of effect} \times \textit{Size of study}$$

A moment's pause with this equation reveals that, obtaining statistical significance is a trivially simple undertaking. As long as the size of the effect is not exactly equal to zero, statistical significance is *guaranteed* as long as the size of the study is large enough. For these and other reasons, reliance on p values and null hypothesis significance testing as a way of progressing science has a long history of criticism. An expanded consideration of that history is not necessary for our current purposes but sources such as Sullivan and Feinn (2012) provide useful introductions.

One of the classic portrayals of the deficiencies of null hypothesis significance testing, and the ceaseless march of p values, comes from Cohen (1994) who exhorts that, the primary problem of our devotion to null hypothesis significance testing is that "it does not tell us what we want to know, and we so much want to know what we want to know that, out of desperation, we nevertheless believe that it does!" (p. 997). According to Cohen (1994), what researchers want to know is, "given the data I have just collected, what is the probability that the null hypothesis is true"? What the null hypothesis significance test tells us, however, is "given that the null hypothesis is true, what is the probability of obtaining these (or more extreme) data"? These two statements are not the same (Cohen, 1994, p. 997). Significance testing is a very low bar upon which to base the progress of a science.

Life Is Not an Averaged Event

Since statistical methods have been, almost exclusively, the tools adopted to grow our knowledge and understanding of health inequity, it is entirely understandable, that aggregated data would be the fodder we gather to fuel our results-generating processes. Wilkinson and Pickett (2018, p. 154), for example, report that "although the role of luck shows us the unpredictability of individual lives, it impinges little on our understanding of average or *group* differences among large populations". Babones (2008, p. 1615) acknowledges that "A difficulty in interpreting the plethora of results based on panels of limited geographical and temporal scope is that the effects of inequality may be inconsistent over samples and periods".

Marmot, Shipley, and Rose (1984) provide a specific description of some of the methodological strategies that are employed when dealing with aggregated data. In their study, they considered the grades of employment of men who had been classified into the groups of administrative, professional, executive, clerical, and "other". They report that "In our earlier analysis, mortality of the executive grades did not differ from that in the professional grade. These two grades are therefore considered together" (p. 1003) even though they also confess that the "professional grades include men of diverse status" (p. 1003).

Other researchers demonstrate a greater appreciation of the importance of the individual experience. Saunders (2010, p. 117), for example, points to the problems that occur when "Whether it be mental illness rates, homicide rates or obesity rates, the authors appeal to *average* differences between countries to support their argument that *every-one* would be better off if incomes were more equally distributed". The deeply personalised nature of individual expectations is especially important to dwell on for our purposes and is supported by existing authorities. Some of the words from Gilbert (2016) that we provided in Chapter 2 are worth repeating here. Gilbert's (2016, p. 70) unambiguous position is that the proposition that our personal security, satisfaction, and self-esteem all hinge on where our "household income is positioned relative to a nebulous group of others exemplifies a narrow materialistic assessment of human nature which denies the diverse motives, ambitions, desires, and beliefs that animate people's lives". In Chapter 3, we also referred to the fact that Gilbert (2016) reminds us that the practical significance (as opposed to the statistical significance) of income inequity can only be judged with respect to the impact it has on people's lives. And a life is always an individual affair regardless of how socially engaged and involved that individual might be. In Chapter 2, we again deferred to Gilbert's (2016) sobering advice that trust and a sense of fairness are "states of mind that are difficult to separate from the context in which they are experienced" (p. 80). A "state of mind" is exclusively an individual experience. Bartley (2017) also indicates an appreciation of the importance of the individual when she points to the confusion that exists when researchers study populations but then seek to apply their findings to health inequity which "exists between groups of individuals in a single society" (p. 119).

Living does not proceed in the aggregate. As we will explain below, understanding the rates at which various things either do or do not occur is unquestionably a valuable pursuit. When calculating these rates occurs to the exclusion of a focus on individuals, however, they can be more misleading than enlightening. Blampied (1999) muses that although the direction of inference in statistical analyses is *always* from the sample to the population, what we often most want to know about is the impact on an individual. That is, frequently our interest is in the exact *opposite* direction from the methods we use to satisfy that interest.

Causality, with respect to social living, is not an aggregated event, and the concept of "public" health can only ever be useful in the most abstract of ways. Health is only ever an individual affair. We need a much greater focus on accurately and precisely understanding individuals and then building up our understanding of relationships, groups, and communities based on that understanding. This might be considered the "Lego" model building approach to progressing our knowledge of social living. Currently, however, our efforts are, almost without exception, the exact reverse. We're building castles in the clouds and then peering down to see if we can assist individuals in their daily busyness of life. The preponderance of available evidence would indicate that the monopolisation of that game plan has been of little long-term value. Perhaps it has been of value to the careers of researchers and decision-makers but it would be hard to mount a compelling argument that it has been of substantial value to the lives of the people who are supposed to be the ultimate beneficiaries of this knowledge-generating industry.

Making It Matter

A suggestion that we offer both explicitly and implicitly throughout this book is that some things matter, and some things don't. Of course, what we haven't explicitly stated until this point is that, once again, the "mattering" of an event, process, or item, is entirely relative. The "it depends" attitude that we referred to in Chapter 3 is especially pertinent here. Does it matter that, in the health inequity sphere, we currently have a very low bar for what counts as scientific acceptability? Does it matter that there is a very strong possibility that the great majority of cutting-edge knowledge, research, and expertise in the inequity universe is based on the wrong model of causality and an incorrect understanding of how people function? Does it matter that, in the behavioural sciences, even though being considered a science seems important, we don't really have widely agreed and accepted standards of right and wrong or correct and incorrect when it comes to judging theories and models? Does it matter that the inequity field is plagued by imprecision, inaccuracy, disagreement, and questionable decision-making processes? Does it matter that, in the shadow of all of these deficiencies, research continues to be funded with tax payers' money, papers and books continue to be published, policies continue to be developed and re-developed, and academic and research careers continue to sprout and blossom?

In a way, we suspect, these questions might have that annoying rhetorical ring about them, as though we are backing you into a conceptual corner and setting you up to provide a *particular* answer. Once the trap has been set and we've snared the answer we want, we can pounce on you with a "See, I told you so" expression and a smug smile. And in a way, you'd be correct. But in another, very important way, there is not a skerrick of rhetoricity in any of these questions. These questions clearly matter to us. What we don't know is if they matter *to you*. So, in that sense, they are not rhetorical at all.

We think it matters to get things right. We think being precise and accurate is the most certain way of getting things right. We also think that now, more than ever before, we have the technology to build a body of knowledge that is oodles more accurate and precise—and ultimately more helpful—than we previously thought possible. We would love to see the iconic words of Feynman that we referred to in Chapter 3, "If it disagrees with experiment, it's wrong", adopted routinely throughout the behavioural sciences. The simple experiments produced in Chapter 3 would be a good starting point. We would relish the introduction of a standard that insists on subjecting any ideas or explanations about how something works or arises to the process of functional model building. Then, the data generated by the model could be compared to the data generated by the phenomenon being explained as the ultimate test of the veracity of one's assumptions.

Most of all, we would be delighted if we were held accountable to these high standards as well. This book is as much a process of organising our own thinking on this topic so we can be clearer about what to do next. We have critically and sceptically committed to understanding living things as control systems. We are also aware, however, that our work does not always reflect that commitment as well as it could. Since completing the equivalent of the transition from a geocentric to a heliocentric understanding of the solar system in our own thinking, we have still had to maintain work routines and schedules, publish papers, work with colleagues, teach and supervise students, and do all the other things that are necessary to hold down a job and maintain our preferred standards of living. This book is as much an evolving manual of how we could be doing more of what we want to do (and less of the things we know are ineffective and inaccurate), as it is an invitation to find more friends and colleagues to do it with.

We have made tremendous progress in many areas … we can send people into outer space, we can build skyscrapers that disappear into the clouds, and bridges that span vast distances. We have also identified, and found ways to successfully combat, tiny itty bitty creatures that can cause devastating illnesses and death on widespread scales. Despite these amazing accomplishments, we still find it hard to get on with each other on a daily basis. Every day in Australia more than 8 people kill themselves. Every other day between 1 and 2 people are killed by someone else.

Premature and unnecessary deaths are tragic but also serious are the many, many lives that are wasted or unfulfilled because of misery and distress generally, or the chaotic, impoverished, or sometimes dangerous environments people live in.

In terms of the ways we treat ourselves and each other, we could be doing much better.

> *There is more than enough evidence to suggest that it might be useful to step back, consider different perspectives, and to ask how we could be doing things differently.* (Carey, 2019)

Solving inequity matters. It also matters that we know what it is about inequity that makes it a problem which needs to be solved. It matters that people, on a large scale, are not living lives they value. We suspect, that if we asked a very large assemblage of the world's population,

Are you living the life you want?

and

Are you able to live the life you want?

we would be disappointed, but perhaps not surprised, by the answers. These two simple questions might provide somewhat of a manifesto for building a body of work that matters and makes a difference.

What Could We Be Studying?

Control matters. The focus of all of our research needs to be underpinned by a model of negative feedback control. We need to study goals, networks of hierarchies of goals, and the environments that help or hinder them. We need our efforts to be informed by an accurate and precise understanding of the way in which goals function in control systems.

Behaviour is undeniably important, but we need to change our understanding of what it is. It is not the final outcome in a series of linear events like the last domino to fall. Behaviour *is* the control of perception (Powers, 1973, 2005). Studying behaviour from a control perspective will lead to different possibilities and more accurate and precise methods of helping people and even knowing when to help and when to get out of the way.

Whether we believe the world is flat or the world is round, we will still see ships sail out to sea and disappear over the horizon. Whether we believe the Earth or the Sun is at the centre of the solar system, we will still refer to "sunsets" and "sunrises", and marvel at their beauty with the appropriate articulation of "Oohs" and "Aahs". Somehow, naming these phenomena "planetary rotations" just wouldn't have the same effect. Observations don't always change with improvements in understanding.

We need to change our version of what behaviour is, and we need to study it differently. As Experiments 1–5 in Chapter 3 demonstrate, different patterns in behaviour tell us about the different conditions of the environment *as they are experienced by the behaver*. These patterns tell us nothing about the internal organisation of the behaver. If we recorded the arm movements of someone steering a car with power steering, and then recorded arm movements for the same steering tasks in a car without power steering, we would obtain *different* records of movements for the *same* goals, purposes, and outcomes.

What Model Could We Use?

Models matter. The models we use, either implicitly or explicitly, inform the questions we ask, and the answers we seek. We are analogue not digital creatures. "One's life is not a succession of actions; but a ceaseless maintenance of one direction and another, a ceaseless pursuit of goals" (Runkel, 2003, p. 19).

Identifying the "start" of a particular process or event is an arbitrary verdict that reveals more about the identifier and what is important to them, than it exposes about the phenomenon under scrutiny. Inequity is often identified at the beginning of some causal sequence affecting variables such as trust or health (Rothstein & Uslaner, 2005; Wilkinson & Pickett, 2010), but this is incorrect. What, for example, should we identify as the starting event or idea that caused the book you are now reading to be produced? Was it when we signed the book contract? A lot had happened before that. Was it the first time we encountered some information about health inequity? How did we come to "encounter" it, and why were we interested enough to find out more? Where do we stop? What was the beginning? We can stop, basically, wherever we want because there is no beginning. The beginning can be where we want it to be depending on our purposes and what we want to demonstrate.

Tangible working models matter, and it is the negative feedback loop that makes models of autonomous, organic control work (Runkel, 2003). We can't have it both ways. "Living creatures do not loop on Mondays and straight-line on Tuesdays. They do not turn the page with loops while reading the print in linear cause-to-effect episodes" (Runkel, 2003, p. 213).

Models matter. Explanations matter. The models we use to inform our cerebrations and practices should be functional models.

What Methods Could We Employ?

Methods matter. There is a well-known adage which proposes that when the only tool you have is a hammer, you are likely to see everything as a nail. This is known as the Law of the Instrument. The idea is especially relevant in the health inequity area. For all practical purposes, in the field of health inequity, there appears to be an almost complete reliance on quantitative methods. A great proportion of these methods are focussed on large samples and association techniques, such as some variation or derivative of correlation or regression.

The choice of method to be used must be driven by the question being asked. Finding answers to a question such as "What is the meaning of having low control at home?" (Chandola et al., 2004, p. 1503) might seem like an important and useful thing to do. Chandola et al. (2004) presented this question at the end of the Introduction of their paper as the first of six questions the research they conducted sought to answer. In this study, however, answers to the meaning of the control question were only sought quantitatively. It was explained in the Data Analysis section that "Two types of analyses were carried out. The first analysed predictors of low control at home using logistic regression and the second analysed the incidence of [coronary heart disease] events as the outcome of a Cox proportional hazards survival analysis" (Chandola et al., 2004, p. 1504). We would argue that a matter such as "meaning" cannot be adequately or meaningfully answered by scores on a self-report questionnaire or some other data generating device from the quantitative arsenal. As we mentioned above, Gilbert (2016) reminds us of the importance of considering the impact on people's lives as well as concepts that should be regarded as "states of mind". Similarly, if we genuinely want to understand the impact of our neighbour's successes on our own well-being, we need to do something other than interrogate massive data sets of artificially constructed residential areas as occurred in the study we referred to in Chapter 2 (Luttmer, 2004). Methods other than the hammer of large sample quantitative methods would be very useful to help unriddle these topics.

In a discussion of methods, it is very much a case of "and" not "or". It may be that, for any particular empirical investigation, a singular method is more appropriate than another discrete method or even multiple methods. A decision such as this, however, should be determined by the research question being asked and not the particular technique the researcher most likes to use. Of course, even in this discussion, the dangerous spectre of linear causality is never far away. The research question being asked will, indubitably, be framed by the researcher who will, in all probability, be the one leading the analysis of the data that are collected. Even in this micro-examination we have returned to the primacy of goals—the researcher's goals. We began this chapter with a discussion of the controlling natures of researchers. Those points are relevant again here.

We unreservedly do not recommend throwing the baby out with the bathwater. Nor do we endorse, however, the automatic assumption that, if there is bathwater which needs to be dispensed, there is necessarily a baby somewhere in there that needs saving. Sometimes, bathwater is just bathwater. Runkel's (1990) canny and perceptive advice is just as relevant now as it was 30 years ago. The title of Runkel's (1990) text describes two "grand methods" for conducting research as "casting nets" and "testing specimens". Both methods, according to Runkel (1990), are necessary for an accurate, precise, and complete empirical and scientific approach to the study of life. The methods incorporated within the casting nets category are essential for understanding the rates at which various things occur, how many of them there are, and so on. Examples of studies that use a casting nets approach, Runkel (1990) argues, would include polling, correlations, and causal experiments. While undoubtedly valuable for answering certain kinds of questions, these methods are *inappropriate* for *explaining* why the phenomena that have been counted or measured occur the way they do, or how these phenomena function. Explanations and answers to questions of function need to be sought through a testing specimens approach.

Casting nets is the hammer of inequity research. Currently, we are requiring much more of casting nets techniques than they will ever be able to deliver. We also appear to be ignoring important areas that casting nets approaches cannot elucidate. If we removed from the inequity field, all existing explanations of various aspects of human functioning or compromised functioning developed by methods that were not designed to be explanatory, we would have a sliver of the quantity of information that is currently available. Building a science involves much more than simply borrowing the scientist's toolbox. Scientists' standards of excellence and rigour, and their attitudes to model building, should also be adopted. While it is the case that methods matter, it is the scientific attitude rather than any particular scientific method that is critically decisive (McIntyre,

2019). Once again, Feynman's words are instructive for the appropriate attitudinal stance to adopt: *If it disagrees with experiment, it's wrong.*

The model-fitting approach that was demonstrated in Experiments 1–5 are a phenomenally more exacting test of one's ideas about how something works than current approaches. A simple tracking task might seem a long way away from the complexities of health and well-being but we would argue that the principles involved are the same. And the approach to theorising, model building, and the identification of mechanisms demonstrated in these experiments could definitely be emulated in other work. We could adopt a standard, for example, that required any declaration of a putative mechanism to be accompanied by a proposal of how the mechanism works.

There is also scope, within a paradigm of control, to develop new methods that might be more fit for purpose than some current approaches. Our own research group is developing an interview schedule based on a technique known as the "test for the controlled variable" (Marken, 2014; Runkel, 1990) to help answer questions related to an individual's important preferences and ideal outcomes. The method capitalises on the fact that control systems are compelled to counteract environmental disturbances to goal states. Yin (2013) outlines the way in which the test for the controlled variable can be applied to the investigation of such things as reflexes and reinforcement rates. First, a hypothesis is generated about what an important goal state for a particular individual might be. Next, questions are asked, or scenarios suggested, that should disturb that state. Responses from the participant are analysed in terms of their effect on the disturbance with subsequent confirmation or refutation of the hypothesis. When the interviewer is in a position to systematically predict what the response will be to a particular question or statement, they will be considered to have obtained some evidence with regard to the goal state.

Don't Go Anywhere! We're Not Done Yet ...

Control is the book of life and control matters. So far, we have outlined some of the important ways in which a widespread recognition of control might affect our attitude to research and subsequent research practices. Specific examples of the way in which a closer consideration of control might enhance our research efforts will be outlined in the following chapter.

References

Babones, S. J. (2008). Income inequality and population health: Correlation and causality. *Social Science and Medicine, 66,* 1614–1626.

Baek, S.-H., & Kim, K.-T. (2018). Retesting the income inequality hypothesis: Pooled time-series-cross-section regression with a new statistical case selection method. *Asian Social Work and Policy Review, 12,* 191–199. https://doi.org/10.1111/aswp.12150.

Bartley, M. (2017). *Health inequality: An introduction to concepts, theories and methods* (2nd ed.). Cambridge: Polity Press.

Blampied, N. M. (1999). A legacy neglected: Restating the case for single-case research in cognitive-behaviour therapy. *Behaviour Change, 16*(2), 89–104.

Bracken, M. B. (2013). *Risk, chance, and causation.* New Haven, CT: Yale University Press.

Carey, T. A. (2019, October 16–18). *Understanding health and wellbeing with the science of control: Implications for becoming stronger.* Keynote Presentation at the Western Australia Rural and Remote Mental Health Conference, Albany, Western Australia.

Chandola, T., Kuper, H., Singh-Manoux, A., Bartley, M., & Marmot, M. (2004). The effect of control at home on CHD events in the Whitehall II study: Gender differences in psychosocial domestic pathways to social inequalities in CHD. *Social Science and Medicine, 58,* 1501–1509.

Coe, R. (2002, September 12–14). *It's the effect size, stupid. What effect size is and why it is important.* Paper presented at the Annual Conference of the British Educational Research Association. University of Exeter, England. Accessed 12 September 2020. https://www.leeds.ac.uk/educol/documents/00002182.htm.

Cohen, J. (1994). The Earth is round (p < .05). *American Psychologist, 49*(12), 997–1003.

Gilbert, N. (2016). *Never enough: Capitalism and the progressive spirit.* Oxford: Oxford University Press.

Kennaway, R. (1998). *Population statistics cannot be used for reliable individual prediction.* Unpublished manuscript. Accessed 12 September 2020. http://www.livingcontrolsystems.com/intro_papers/population_stats.pdf.

Luttmer, E. F. P. (2004). *Neighbors as negatives: Relative earnings and well-being* (KSG Working Paper No. RWP04-029). Accessed 12 September 2020. https://papers.ssrn.com/sol3/papers.cfm?abstract_id=571824.

Malkina-Pykh, I., & Pykh, Y. (2019, March 28–30). *Linear vs. nonlinear regression models in psychology and life sciences: Why to compare non-comparable.* 8th International Nonlinear Science Conference. Coimbra, Portugal. https://doi.org/10.13140/rg.2.2.11641.11362. Accessed 12 September 2020.

https://www.researchgate.net/publication/332207546_Linear_vs_Nonlinear_Regression_Models_in_Psychology_and_Life_Sciences_Why_to_Compare_Non-comparable?channel=doi&linkId=5ca607ef4585157bd3219835&showFulltext=true.

Marken, R. S. (2014). *Doing research on purpose: A control theory approach to experimental psychology*. St Louis, MO: New View.

Marmot, M. G., Shipley, M. J., & Rose, G. (1984, May 5). Inequalities in death—Specific explanations of a general pattern? *The Lancet, 323,* 1003–1006.

McIntyre, L. (2019). *The scientific attitude: Defending science from denial, fraud, and pseudoscience*. Cambridge, MA: The MIT Press.

Pearl, J. (2009). Causal inference in statistics: An overview. *Statistics Surveys, 3,* 96–146.

Pickett, K. E., & Wilkinson, R. G. (2015). Income inequality and health: A causal review. *Social Science and Medicine, 128,* 316–326.

Powers, W. T. (1973). *Behavior: The control of perception*. Chicago: Aldine.

Powers, W. T. (1990). Control theory and statistical generalizations. *American Behavioral Scientist, 34*(1), 24–31.

Powers, W. T. (2005). *Behavior: The control of perception* (2nd ed.). New Canaan, CT: Benchmark.

Rosnow, R. L., & Rosenthal, R. (2013). *Beginning behavioral research: A conceptual primer* (7th ed.). Boston: Pearson.

Rothstein, B., & Uslaner, E. M. (2005). All for all: Equality, corruption, and social trust. *World Politics, 58*(1), 41–72.

Runkel, P. J. (1990). *Casting nets and testing specimens: Two grand methods of psychology*. New York: Praeger.

Runkel, P. J. (2003). *People as living things: The psychology of perceptual control*. Hayward, CA: Living Control Systems Publishing.

Saunders, P. (2010). *Beware false prophets: Equality, the good society, and the spirit level*. London: Policy Exchange.

Scambler, G., & Scambler, S. (2015). Theorizing health inequalities: The untapped potential of dialectical critical realism. *Society Theory & Health, 13*(3–4), 340–354.

Schneider, S. M. (2019). Why income inequality is dissatisfying—Perceptions of social status and the inequality-satisfaction link in Europe. *European Sociological Review, 35*(3), 409–430. https://doi.org/10.1093/esr/jcz003.

Sullivan, G. M., & Feinn, R. (2012). Using effect size—Or why the *P* value is not enough. *Journal of Graduate Medical Education, 4*(3), 279–282. https://doi.org/10.4300/JGME-D-12-00156.1.

Wilkinson, R., & Pickett, K. (2010). *The spirit level: Why equality is better for everyone*. London: Penguin Books.

Wilkinson, R., & Pickett, K. (2018). *The inner level: How more equal societies reduce stress, restore sanity and improve everyone's well-being*. London: Penguin Random House.

Yin, H. H. (2013). Restoring purpose in behavior. In G. Baldassarre & M. Mirolli (Eds.), *Computational and robotic models of the hierarchical organization of behaivor* (pp. 319–347). London: Springer.

CHAPTER 7

Yes! That Really *Is* What We Mean

We have to live today by what truth we can get today, and be ready tomorrow to call it falsehood. William James

So far throughout the book, we have outlined some general principles and concepts that could, potentially, transform the health inequity domain in terms of understanding and impact. At the end of the previous chapter, we began to sketch out some of our initial ideas for how we might advance the study of inequity. In these next two chapters, we'd like to build on this sketch and provide some more specific ideas about where a new approach might lead. In this chapter, we'll concentrate on research and in the next chapter we'll consider ideas for health professionals and other practitioners.

Researching Controllers

To illustrate some of the possibilities for the way in which research might change, we're going to focus on a specific study that has already been published. We learned about this work while we were ploughing through the health inequity field. It's important for us to emphasise at the outset, that our comments, ideas, and suggestions are not intended to be rebukes of this research. Indeed, we selected this article because of how interesting and important we think the study is. Our only disappointment with the

T. A. Carey et al., *Deconstructing Health Inequity*,
https://doi.org/10.1007/978-3-030-68053-4_7

research we are considering is that it is replete with unfulfilled potential. What we intend to demonstrate throughout this chapter is how an understanding of ourselves and our research participants as controllers could help to enrich and refine programmes of research so that a more accurate and precise portrayal is delivered of that bit of human functioning with which the research is concerned. To that end, we don't intend to dissect every single detail of this study. Rather, our aim is to focus attention on those aspects of the study that are especially relevant from a control perspective. These areas of relevance are the points at which an alternative way of thinking might have produced different outcomes and conclusions for the project.

The paper we focus on in this chapter is an experimental study from 2004 by Hoff and Pandey. The paper is titled *Belief systems and durable inequalities: An experimental investigation of Indian caste* and was published as World Bank Policy Research Working Paper 3351.

The paper was absorbing to us for several reasons. It's an interesting study in an important area of social relationships. It demonstrates many of the points we've raised throughout the previous chapters and it provides some tantalising suggestions for how an understanding of people as controllers might have extended and improved both the research and the conclusions. In the following sections, we provide the impressions, ideas, and suggestions that occurred to us as we tracked through the paper.

Setting the Scene: Detecting Clues About Control from the Very Beginning

To establish the justification for the study, Hoff and Pandey (2004) begin with a brief statement about the economic impact of colonisation in regions where Europe had maintained a colonial presence. It is suggested that "economists have emphasized that the past shapes opportunities – for example, the security of property rights, the level of literacy, and the distribution of wealth – which shape the economy" (Hoff & Pandey, 2004, p. 3). Hoff and Pandey, however, propose another explanation, the test of which is the research they conduct and describe. Hoff and Pandey (2004, p. 3) suggest that "the past shapes belief systems that shape individuals' *response* to opportunities" and that "the expectations that historical conditions created may remain and give rise to behaviors that reproduce the effects of those historical barriers".

From the beginning, therefore, Hoff and Pandey (2004) signal their allegiance to the linear model of causality in which certain behaviours or responses are "shaped" by events that precede them. They also illustrate their subscription to a third-person perspective of understanding and investigating behaviour. We were encouraged by the mention of "expectations", but we didn't really expect that a PCT depiction of expectations would appear.

Hoff and Pandey (2004) go on to explain that they intend to "experimentally test the hypothesis that belief systems that are the legacy of historical conditions of extreme inequality give rise to expectations of prejudicial treatment and hence to behaviours that tend to reproduce the inequality" (p. 4). In this statement, Hoff and Pandey implicitly communicate some of the meta-method assumptions which guide their work. Statements such as this also provide evidence of their own functioning as control systems in terms of the result they seek to produce (testing a hypothesis). Figure 7.1 provides a schematic diagram that is our interpretation of the model Hoff and Pandey seemed to be describing.

Remarkably, even here there is a whiff of an idea that could quickly and easily metamorphosise into a control system model if Hoff and Pandey (2004) had understood the actual phenomenon with which they were dealing. Figure 7.2 is a tentative and preliminary depiction of the model that might inform our investigations were we to undertake a study of this kind. Even a cursory inspection of this model suggests different questions that would become important such as: what are the controlled variable aspects of the environment that correspond to the hypothesised belief systems and expectations; what environmental factors help or hinder control of these variables; and how do these goal states relate to other important goal states of the individual?

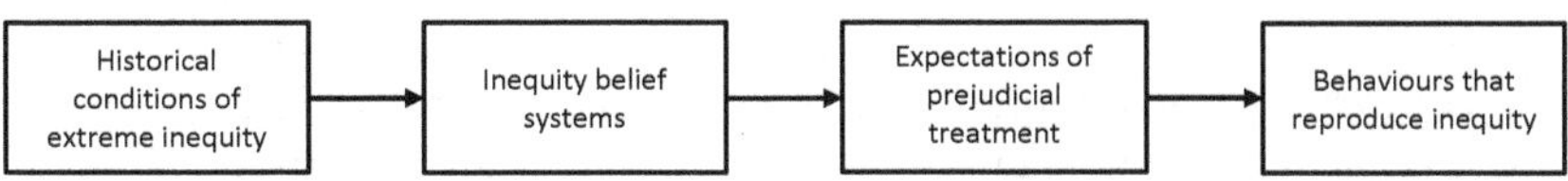

Fig. 7.1 Our interpretation of the model informing Hoff and Pandey's (2004) experimental work

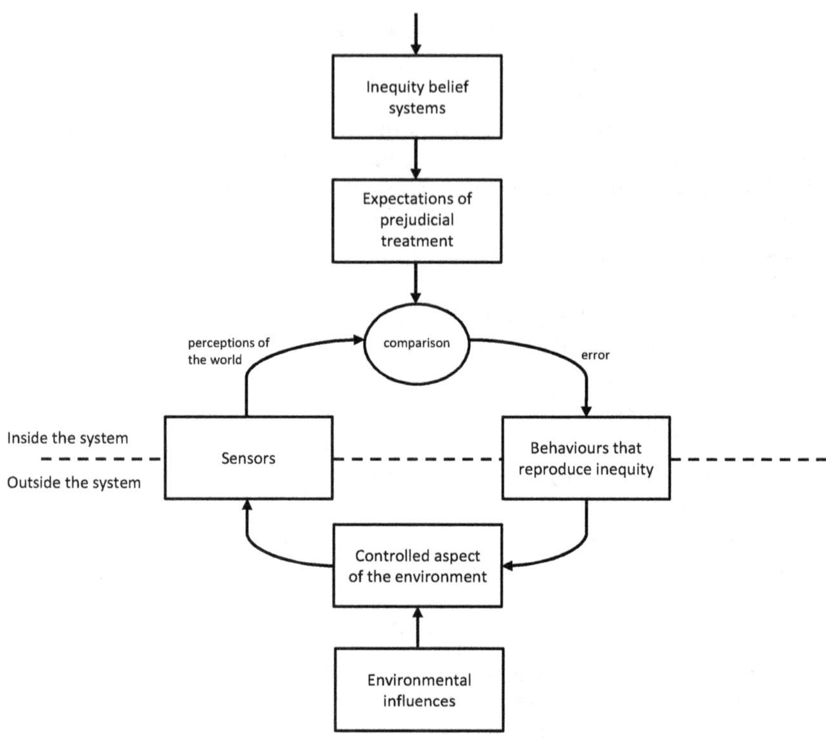

Fig. 7.2 A model depicting a hierarchical, control system organisation of the subject matter described by Hoff and Pandey (2004)

The Controllers Who Made It Happen

If we accept that people are controllers, then, in order to understand the study accurately and precisely, the activity of all of the people involved should be considered. The controlling of the authors of the study, Hoff and Pandey, for example, could be explored. Then, there were the people who completed the activities designed by Hoff and Pandey, as well as other people who were mentioned, such as the graders of the mazes, the assistants who supervised the participants while they were waiting, and the parents of the participants (Hoff & Pandey, 2004).

Hoff and Pandey

The controlling of Hoff and Pandey as the designers of the study and the authors of the publication is clearly important to consider. The conceptualisation of the project, the outcomes that were achieved, and the way in which the outcomes were reported were all aspects of Hoff and Pandey's controlling. On the publication, Hoff's affiliation is stated to be the World Bank whereas Pandey's is Pennsylvania State University. Although the study was published in 2004, Hoff's affiliation still appears to be the World Bank. Pandey's current affiliation, however, is more difficult to ascertain.

The available evidence indicates that this was an important study for both Hoff and Pandey. For example, in an interview on the ideas42 website dated April 17, 2018, Hoff refers to this study and its importance to her career.[1] With regard to Pandey, information provided on pages 6 and 7 (which we will return to soon) indicates that she is an educated Indian woman who is "recognizably high caste" (p. 6). The significance of Pandey's background will become clearer below. It appears, also, that Pandey took an active role in the study. We learn on page 7 that "The experiment was almost double-blind – the Experimenters (except Pandey) did not know the hypotheses of the study, and the graders of the mazes did not know the castes of the subjects".

It may be unnecessary to clarify that "almost double-blind" is not double-blind at all. What is of more interest, however, to our analysis, is the fact that Hoff and Pandey (2004) ensured this information was provided to readers. We might speculate about what intended outcomes Hoff and Pandey (2004) were controlling by communicating to readers that their study was "almost double-blind". What might they have wanted readers to think about their study? Could they, perhaps, have been interested in asserting a certain level of rigour, credibility, and persuasiveness to the research?

Experimenters

In this paper, Hoff and Pandey (2004) appear to refer to the staff who ran the experiments as "Experimenters". Little information is provided about these experimenters. It is explained that "The site of the

[1] https://www.ideas42.org/blog/ideas42-seminar-series-talk-karla-hoff/.

experiment was a junior high school in a village in central Uttar Pradesh, India. We recruited from cities in Uttar Pradesh a staff to run the experiments. Being educated Indian women, the Experimenters were recognizably high caste" (Hoff & Pandey, 2004, p. 6). As mentioned above, it is stated that the Experimenters (apart from Pandey) were unaware of the hypotheses of the study. We are not provided, however, with any information regarding the way in which the Experimenters were recruited. We know they were educated and high caste (Hoff & Pandey, 2004). Were they also employed? Were they paid to participate as Experimenters? Did they have to take time off from their regular employment? What was their interest in participating in the study if they were unaware of the hypotheses of the study? Whereas the Experimenters were recruited from cities in Uttar Pradesh, the study was conducted at "a junior high school in a village in central Uttar Pradesh" (Hoff & Pandey, 2004, p. 6). How were the Experimenters, therefore, transported to the study site?

Participants and Parents

Hoff and Pandey (2004) explain that it was a "challenge to find representative subjects who would feel comfortable in a classroom setting" (p. 7), although they don't explain what representative criteria they used or why a classroom setting was necessary. In footnote number 14 at the bottom of page 7, Hoff and Pandey (2004) provide the following information: "we are not aware of any selection factors that make the children who were drawn from the 6th and 7th grades unrepresentative of all 11-12 year olds. In particular, in the schools we visited, children appeared to be automatically promoted to the next grade level each year". This information didn't address our queries regarding representativeness. We did think, however, that it was further interesting information for Hoff and Pandey (2004) to communicate in terms of the impression of the research they might have wanted readers to form.

The particulars about the recruitment procedure are scant, but Hoff and Pandey (2004, p. 7) are clear that they "chose as subjects 6th and 7th -graders". Furthermore, they "recruited boys from the lowest caste, Chamar, and the three highest castes: Thakur, Brahmin, and Vaishya, which respectively constituted 70, 24, and 6 percent of the high-caste subjects" (Hoff & Pandey, 2004, p. 7). In footnote number 15 at the bottom of page 7, Hoff and Pandey report that:

> *Throughout most of the period of the experiment, schools were closed. To recruit children, we visited homes each evening to ask parents' permission to pick up their children the next day to drive them to the nearby junior high school that served as the site of the experiment. We told the parents that participants would be paid for showing up and additional rewards depending on performance. We stated that our purpose was to study children in India. In only a few instances, parents refused to let their children participate, and the reason was that their neighbor was angry that we had not paid him money for driving his child to the junior high school instead of letting us transport the child.*

We are not entirely sure what is being communicated in the last sentence, however, it seems clear that financial considerations were at least partly involved in some of the decision-making that occurred during the research process. The impact that monetary matters had on the research is unable to be determined, however, it may well have been considerable. Hoff and Pandey (2004, p. 7) explain that "At the beginning of an experimental session, the Experimenter gave participants the show-up fee of 10 rupees (a significant amount compared to the 6 rupee unskilled adult hourly wage) to drive home the fact that the children were playing for money".

In addition to the show-up fee, there was the opportunity for children to obtain more money depending on the number of mazes they solved. On page 8, further details are provided about these extra finances. "Not counting the show-up fee, the top performers earned 2.2 times a day's unskilled wages in a session that lasted about one hour. Average earnings were slightly less than one-half a day's wages. Each subject participated in only one session" (Hoff & Pandey, 2004). In addition to what could be earned for showing up and solving mazes we are informed that "To promote trust, participants received a piece of fruit on entering the room of the experiment, a 'consolation prize' of two rupees if they solved no mazes, and full awards to all winners who tied in a tournament" (Hoff & Pandey, 2004, p. 8). Given the finances involved, therefore, it is at least possible that the amount of money being provided might have influenced the goals, priorities, and preferences of the children who participated and even their parents. Yet there was no discussion of this possible influence throughout the paper.

Other People Who Were Involved in the Research

It is not clear how many other people were involved in the research, how they were recruited, what they might have been paid, or the potential they might have had to influence the project. In footnote number 18 at the bottom of page 8, we learn that "Our assistants maintained a peaceful atmosphere in the school courtyard where children waited to participate in the experiment or to be paid. Parents of the children were free to wait there, too. Our assistant distributed box lunches at midday" (Hoff & Pandey, 2004). It is also stated that people referred to as "graders" were involved in the study, however, there are few details about them. All we are told is that "the graders of the mazes did not know the castes of the subjects" (Hoff & Pandey, 2004, p. 8). We also discover on page 8 that "As soon as the mazes from an experimental session were graded (normally within two hours), the earnings were distributed in sealed envelopes to the participants, who were asked not to open them until they returned home" (Hoff & Pandey, 2004). The graders, therefore, seem likely to have been situated at the same site as the experiment. So, presumably, participants waited in the courtyard with a peaceful atmosphere for up to two hours to discover how much more money, apart from the 10 rupees, they were going to take home. While they were waiting, they were likely to have been in the company of other children who were yet to participate.

The Procedures and Activities

The project consisted of a number of discrete experiments. For our purposes, what was of most interest were the instructions given and any clues about what the goals of all the contributors and participants to each experiment might have been. On pages 2 and 3, Hoff and Pandey (2004) provide an overview of the project:

> *We have groups of six male junior high school students perform the task of solving mazes. Three experimental conditions provide a contrast in the salience of caste. In the first condition, caste is not publicly revealed. In the second condition, the Experimenter publicly announces the caste of each subject. In the third condition, groups consist of only high-caste individuals or only low-caste ("Untouchable") individuals and, as in the preceding case, the Experimenter publicly announces caste.*

Although this description seems straightforward, the actual descriptions of the studies were less clear. In the section titled "Experiment 1: Caste and Performance", for example, the objective is described as being "to determine whether increasing the salience of caste changes the ability or propensity of low-caste subjects to respond to economic incentives" (p. 6). As an aside, we should point out the obvious meta-method presumption of linear causality being communicated here. In terms of furthering our understanding of what occurred, it is stated that participants in this experiment "were asked to solve mazes in two 15-minute rounds" (p. 6).

The description of the conditions of the research on pages 2 and 3 (Hoff & Pandey, 2004) has no easily discernible direct connection with the studies that are subsequently described. For example, the paper has four general sections: I—A short background on the caste system; II—Experiment 1: Caste and performance; III—Experiment 2: Manipulating the scope for Experimenter discretion; and IV—Conclusion. Within Section II, six subsections labelled A to F are outlined. It is in these subsections that the main studies are described, and it is here that we focus our attention.

The Variables and Treatments

In what appears to be the main body of work, the number of mazes solved in each round is described as the primary dependent variable (Hoff & Pandey, 2004). As mentioned earlier, it was stated that Experimenters provided the show-up fee of 10 rupees at the beginning of each experimental session "to drive home the fact that the children were playing for money" (Hoff & Pandey, 2004, p. 7). As independent variables, Hoff and Pandey (2004) describe "varying whether or not we announced caste", "the incentive systems across treatments", and "the caste composition of the group" (p. 9).

The different treatments are listed in Table 1 (Hoff & Pandey, 2004, p. 33). There are eight different treatment conditions described, with caste being announced in six of them. Every treatment was conducted with groups of six boys per testing and, in seven of the treatments, the groups consisted of three high-caste and three low-caste boys. The total number of participants in each treatment condition varied from 60 to 120. Overall, there were 107 sessions with 642 participants (Hoff & Pandey, 2004).

The Treatment Instructions

The instructions for each experimental condition are provided in an appendix at the end of the paper. The instructions clearly emphasise how much money participants will receive for their involvement in the study. In some of the treatments, the total amount that a participant could receive is substantial. For example, in Treatment 2, labelled the "Mixed Tournament" treatment, it is explained that "only one child will get a reward. The child who gets the reward is the one who solves the greatest number of puzzles" (Hoff & Pandey, 2004, p. 41). In addition to the instructions which were read out (it was explained that it was decided to read out all instructions due to literacy problems), a table was provided to illustrate one possible scenario. There is no number or title for the table, but it is step "10-T" of the section "2. Mixed Tournament" on page 41 (Hoff & Pandey, 2004).

The explanation accompanying this table is: "The winner would be Geeta. She solved the largest number of puzzles. And she would get 36 rupees. No other child would get any money. *Experimenter checks that each child understands the reward system by changing one or two numbers in the table and then asking him what the rewards would be*" (Hoff & Pandey, 2004, p. 41). We find it curiously unfathomable that Hoff and Pandey would devise a study with exclusively low- and high- caste 11- and 12-year-old males, being guided through the activities by recognisably high-caste females and, in that context, provide an example to explain one of the activities by depicting a female winning all the rupees. In the circumstances of the activities, the male participants were undertaking, that scenario would have been impossible. We're puzzled as to what Hoff and Pandey (2004) intended to communicate with this particular illustration, and we also wonder what the experience of the boys might have been in being presented with this scenario.

In the conditions in which caste was announced, it is reported that "the Experimenter turned to each participant and stated his name, village, father's and grandfather's names, and caste and asked him to nod if the information was correct" (Hoff & Pandey, 2004, p. 12). Although this is the only information provided about the announcement of caste, it is further stated that this condition was designed to "investigate whether announcing social identity (caste) affects performance" (Hoff & Pandey, 2004, p. 12), to "determine whether increasing the salience of caste changes ability or propensity of low-caste subjects to respond to economic incentives" (p. 6), and to explore "the way individuals adapt when they know the Experimenter, knows and is concerned, with their caste membership" (p. 8). Given that the only information we have is the instructions read out by the Experimenters, it is not clear how Hoff and Pandey (2004) were able to ascertain that caste had been made "salient" for every boy, or how they determined that the boys thought the Experimenters were "concerned" about their caste membership.

The Results

Generally, it seems reasonable to conclude that the results occurred the way Hoff and Pandey (2004) expected them to. Or, perhaps more accurately, Hoff and Pandey (2004) organised and reported the results in a way that was consistent with what their expectations appeared to be. Reviewing the numbers with perhaps a different expectation, however, reveals some possible anomalies.

Hoff and Pandey (2004) report that "caste is irrelevant to performance when caste is not announced" (p. 10). Interestingly, Hoff and Pandey (2004) present many of their results in tables as cumulative percentages although there is no explanation given as to why the results are presented in this way. Here, then, is another example of researchers, in the process of their controlling, making decisions to achieve intended results (the way they present their findings) even though we might not know what those intentions are.

A further example of Hoff and Pandey's (2004) controlling is provided when they report the results of the experiments in which each of the boys' caste is announced. Hoff and Pandey (2004) describe the effect of this announcement as "debilitating" for the low-caste boys. Hoff and Pandey refer to Figure 2 (2004, p. 13) to provide evidence of this "debilitating" effect. Once again, the figure provides cumulative percentages. A debilitating effect is not immediately apparent to us from inspecting Figure 2, and nor is it discernible to us from the means and standard deviations that can be extracted from Table 3 (Hoff & Pandey, 2004, p. 35). Perhaps we have a different understanding of "debilitating" to the understanding Hoff and Pandey (2004) intended to communicate. Although only the means are provided in the text on page 13, standard deviations are also provided in Table 3 (Hoff & Pandey, 2004, p. 35). We have distilled the relevant data here, and presented them in Table 7.1, so that we can more carefully consider the labelling of a "debilitating effect". We would

Table 7.1 Means and standard deviations extracted from Table 3 of Hoff and Pandey (2004, p. 35) which relates to the information they describe on page 13. The range of scores that represents one standard deviation above and below each of the means is also reported

Caste	Statistics	Caste Not Announced (n = 96)	Caste Announced (n = 120)
High	Mean	5.54	6.11
	Standard Deviation (SD)	3.93	3.42
	Mean +/- 1 SD	1.61 – 9.47	2.69 – 9.53
Low	Mean	5.72	4.28
	Standard Deviation (SD)	3.52	3.20
	Mean +/- 1 SD	2.20 – 9.24	1.08 – 7.48

regard the discovery of a "debilitating effect" for 11- and 12-year-old boys in the context of having their caste announced to be a remarkable and noteworthy finding. Table 7.1, however, indicates that "debilitating" might not be the most appropriate descriptor to have chosen. We wonder what Hoff and Pandey's (2004) intentions might have been when they selected this particular word to use.

The information we are presenting here is not intended to contradict or criticise Hoff and Pandey (2004). Instead, we simply wish to highlight, that the set of results from practically any study can be organised in various ways depending on the message that the researchers wish to convey. The message communicated will have everything to do with what the researchers are controlling for in terms of the goals that are important to them. The reason we have included a row in Table 7.1 that describes the range of scores that would fall within one standard deviation above and below each mean is merely to spotlight the amount of overlap there is within the set of scores. It is undeniably the case that many low-caste boys will have completed more correct mazes than high-caste boys in both experiments, regardless of whether caste was or was not announced (see Fig. 7.3).

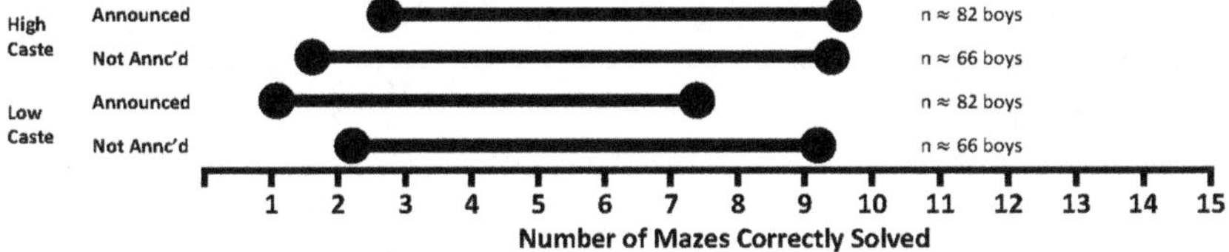

Fig. 7.3 A graphical illustration of the amount of overlap between the groups for the 68.27% of boys who were one standard deviation above or below the mean of number of mazes correctly solved

Table 7.2 Means of number of mazes solved rounded to whole numbers

Caste	Statistics	Caste Not Announced (n = 96)	Caste Announced (n = 120)
High	Mean	6.00	6.00
Low	Mean	6.00	4.00

Unlike, Hoff and Pandey (2004), we do not see "debilitation" here. It is clearly the case that a change occurred from the experiment when caste was not announced, to the experiment when caste was announced, however, what should be made of that difference, is far less obvious. Furthermore, reporting the number of correct mazes to two decimal places is somewhat misleading given that a maze can only be either correct or incorrect. Table 7.2 demonstrates what the means would be if only whole numbers were reported.

Our intent in providing Table 7.2 for your consideration is only to demonstrate the way in which the same numbers can be used to communicate different messages depending on the drives of the researchers. Numbers don't care what we do with them. We care, on the other hand, because we are controllers. The way in which numbers are reported will depend entirely upon the effects the reporter of the numbers wishes to create.

It is also worth flagging that the numbers we report, from Hoff and Pandey's (2004, p. 35) Table 7.2, are provided by different groups of boys. As our Tables 7.1 and 7.2 indicate, the data we have used from Hoff and Pandey's Table 3 (p. 35) indicate that one set of means was calculated on a sample of 96 boys and the other set of means was calculated on a sample of 120 boys. The implications this has for the conclusions that are reported will, once again, be tempered by the controlling habits and inclinations of the reporter.

We do not intend to articulate the same level of scrutiny to all the results provided by Hoff and Pandey (2004). Many of the matters we have already raised about the problems with aggregated data and the limitations of significance testing are amply demonstrated in Hoff and Pandey's (2004) work. Before leaving this section, however, one more result is worth signalling in terms of the way in which it is reported.

Apparently, "Among subjects whose scores improved by 5 mazes or more, the fraction of low-caste subjects was 65 percent in the control condition, but 27 percent when caste was announced" (p. 14). Once again, Hoff and Pandey (2004) refer to this as a "debilitating effect". We do not dispute at all that a change from 65% to 27% is noteworthy. What we find even more remarkable, however, is that almost a third of the low-caste boys improved their scores by 5 mazes or more, *after their caste was announced*. Given that there were only 15 mazes to solve, the fact that the maze solving of some low-caste boys *improved* by 5 or more mazes *after* it was revealed to everyone involved in the activity that they were of low-caste origins is something approaching spectacular.

To dwell on this point a little longer, applying these results hypothetically to an individual we have conjured might help to illustrate the enormity of what some boys accomplished. What we understand Hoff and Pandey (2004) to be communicating here is that, if Samesh solved 6 out of 15 mazes in the first experiment, after everyone was told that he was of low-caste he then solved 11 or more mazes. We find this astonishing. We would be very interested in knowing more about the goals, expectations, preferences, values, and controlling habits of Samesh and what we could learn from him. Such learning, however, will be impossible while we cling like limpets to the rock of aggregated data, statistical significance, and the third-person sovereignty of the researcher.

What Is Striking

For us, this study is noteworthy for a number of reasons. The setting, the age of the participants, and the activities are all features that contribute to this being a memorable and important body of work. From a control perspective, however, the number of untested assumptions made throughout the study is one of the most striking features of this research.

Two assumptions were perhaps more about the design of the study. As mentioned above, informing readers that the study was "almost double-blind" seemed important to Hoff and Pandey (2004) yet there was no mention of any checks being conducted to determine if the "almost double-blind" status had been maintained throughout the study. The second assumption related to the design of the study is revealed by Hoff and Pandey (2004, p. 2) when they draw attention to the "controlled experiments" they conduct by explaining that, among other things, structuring the activities in this way enabled them "to measure performance precisely". It is anomalous to us that researchers would emphasise precision as a priority, and yet report only aggregated data. When the phenomenon of interest is human functioning, our stance, as we have indicated previously, is that aggregated data masks, rather than magnifies, precision. Our reservations about the reliance on the use of aggregated statistics (such as means and standard deviations) among those seeking to understand the behaviour of individuals are shared by Arocha (2020), who also questions whether these approaches are truly an effective way to understand such phenomena.

While these two assumptions were important, it was the suppositions about salience and expectations that really grabbed our attention. In particular, salience and expectations appear to be two concepts that are critically central to the study. Regarding salience, for example, determining "whether increasing the salience of caste changes the ability or propensity of low-caste subjects to respond to economic incentives" (Hoff & Pandey, p. 6) was described as an objective of the experiment. Hoff and Pandey (2004) are similarly frank in terms of the importance of expectations to their study when they inform us that "our main conjecture revolves around expectations" (p. 28), and this focus was used as justification for a follow-up study.

We were not at all troubled by the fact that Hoff and Pandey (2004) decided to conduct a study investigating something they called "expectations". We were somewhat perturbed, however, by the fact that important terms like "expectations" and "salience" were never defined, and nor were any efforts described to investigate expectations at their source—that is, to understand the first-person perspective from which expectations manifest. Neither did there seem to be any evidence to verify that caste had in fact become "salient" (however that was defined) and, again, what "salient" might mean to different individuals from a first-person perspective.

Perhaps the most compelling evidence of Hoff and Pandey's (2004) meta-method convictions regarding expectations, as well as their views about what the study demonstrated, is provided in the Conclusion section. Hoff and Pandey (2004, p. 32) explain that:

> *a social identity – a product of history, culture, and personal experience of discrimination – creates a pronounced economic disadvantage for a group through its effect on individuals' expectations. In the experiment, participants had a sociocultural category membership activated by the public announcement of their caste identities and by segregating groups by caste. In controlled settings, in which any possible difference in treatment toward castes was removed, social identity affected behavior largely because it affected expectations. Thus, the findings provide evidence for an additional explanation, beyond differences in access to various resources, for the tendency of social inequalities to reproduce themselves over time.*

And they suggest (Hoff & Pandey, 2004, p. 32):

> *Not only do these findings provide an explanation of the persistence of historical inequalities across social groups, but they also suggest how corrosive the effects can be. In the experiment, activating caste identities debilitated the low caste and hurt even the performance of the high castes.*

In these and similar sentences, Hoff and Pandey (2004) probably do more to communicate some of their own highly valued expectations, preferences, and beliefs about the world than they do to accurately, precisely, and unambiguously portray the outcomes of their research. They completely disregard, for example, the Samesh's of their experiments for whom, we might argue, the evidence suggests were exhilarated, rather than debilitated, by the announcement of their membership of the low-caste club. Hoff and Pandey's (2004) Conclusion section, in fact, could, in many ways, be regarded as a succinct summary of many of the points we have raised so far throughout this book. Their remarks, for example, demonstrate how dangerously brittle inferences about individuals can be when they are based on aggregated data. They also allude to possible mechanistic processes when they describe something or other being "activated". At no stage, however, is there any indication of Hoff and Pandey (2004) subjecting their assumptions to the testing rigours of functional model building.

What Else Is There to Say?

Research is important. If we are to ever use research effectively to resolutely solve some of our most pressing social problems on a scale that is both expansive and enduring, we need to lift our collective game considerably. Control is the game changer.

Science is important. If it's important for us to consider that we are contributing to the scientific enterprise within our field, then we need to focus much more on a scientific *attitude* (McIntyre, 2019) rather than simply going through the motions of apparently scientific routines and procedures.

We need to demand much higher standards for determining the importance or noteworthiness of research findings, as well as far greater precision and accuracy when defining "mechanisms", "causality", and other important scientific dohickeys. Something that Hoff and Pandey (2004) could have changed, for example, would have been the assumption of a linear relationship between the proposed independent and dependent variables. Instead, this would have been replaced by the assumption that everyone involved in the study, researchers, participants, and others is constantly controlling their experiences in line with internally specified reference values that are unique to each of them. At every moment throughout the study, the participants, researchers, and others were counteracting disturbances that would otherwise have disrupted their ability to maintain their experiences in ways that were satisfactory to them. From this angle, rather than changes to participants' performance being understood as a consequence of revealing an individual's caste to others, participants' behaviour would be understood as attempts by those individuals to maintain controlled variables in internally specified states.

Another difference to the design of Hoff and Pandey's (2004) study that would have arisen from the adoption of a PCT frame of mind is its reliance on aggregated data. Runkel's (2007) delineation of two broad categories of research methodology: casting nets and testing specimens, that we introduced earlier, is also relevant here. Hoff and Pandey's (2004) study would fall into the former category. Far more illuminating findings might have been produced, however, if a testing specimens approach had been adopted.

We have demonstrated some of the implications for the conduct of research in the health inequity field of shifting the phenomenon of control to centre stage. Such a shift would also have profound implications for the way in which health services and systems are organised. In the next chapter, we describe what some of these implications are and the way in which health professionals and health system managers might reorient and reorganise their services to improve effectiveness and efficiency. Such efforts can be expected to enhance access to these services and ensure a more equitable distribution of an important but finite resource.

References

Arocha, J. F. (2020). Scientific realism and the issue of variability in behavior. *Theory and Psychology*, 1–24. https://doi.org/10.1177/0959354320935972.

Hoff, K., & Pandey, P. (2004). *Belief systems and durable inequalities: An experimental investigation of Indian Caste* (World Bank Policy Research Working Paper 3351). https://doi.org/10.1596/1813-9450-3351.

McIntyre, L. (2019). *The scientific attitude: Defending science from denial, fraud, and pseudoscience*. Cambridge, MA: The MIT Press.

Runkel, P. J. (2007). *Casting nets and testing specimens* (2nd ed.). Hayward, CA: Living Control Systems Publishing.

CHAPTER 8

But Wait, There's More! Control Affects Practice as Much as Research

I cannot say whether things will get better if we change; what I can say is they must change if they are to get better. George C. Lichtenberg

We are aware that the focus of this book has been heavily weighted towards the body of research and associated commentary that characterises the state of health inequity knowledge. Much less information has been discussed in relation to the implications that a control paradigm has for health professionals and other practitioners who are addressing health inequity "in the field". This imbalance perhaps reflects the areas where we found the largest discrepancies and where our greatest learning occurred. As practising health professionals, we already have some experience in addressing inequity and social justice at an individual, group, and even community level. What we were unprepared for was the dishevelled state of the empirical literature, with inaccurate reporting, disagreements and contradictory findings, as well as implausible and sometimes emotive explanations.

Thus far, therefore, we have provided our impressions of the empirical literature, as well as some ideas we have about what might be done to improve it. In the previous chapter, we focussed specifically on one particular study to illustrate how things might be different in a world where "people as controllers" was understood to be the fact that it is (Marken,

T. A. Carey et al., *Deconstructing Health Inequity*,
https://doi.org/10.1007/978-3-030-68053-4_8

1988). In this chapter, we concentrate on some of the important implications that the fact of organic, autonomous control has for health services and systems as well as clinical practices. In this regard, we are perhaps adding to voices such as Burns (2014) who suggests that health professionals could be contributing to the creation of health rather than simply the treatment and prevention of disease. From our perspective, helping to support the creation of health would first require that health professionals understand health as control (Carey, 2016).

Acknowledging People as Controllers in Our Practices

Accepting that people are controllers, and embracing the ramifications of that, means that the practices of health professionals will never be the same. Health professionals are controllers, their colleagues are controllers, their managers are controllers, their assistants are controllers, their patients are controllers, and their patients' families and carers are controllers. Control is a game that everyone plays. It is a game that everyone *must* play.

A big part of getting comfortable with our controlling nature involves understanding that we all have goals. Not only that, but we have hierarchical networks of goals. We are designed to push back or nullify influences from the environment that nudge our world out of its goal states (Marken & Carey, 2015). Becoming more aware of the goal states, we protect in our work as health professionals can be an important step in improving the efficiency and effectiveness of our efforts. Increasing our awareness of our own and others' controlling propensities provides no guarantee that we'll enjoy a hassle-free workplace ever after. In fact, you might find that, in some areas, you become more perturbed than you were before as you realise that a range of policies and practices in health settings often ride roughshod over the preferences and proclivities of both service providers and service recipients. Health service managers can ignore the goals and values of health professionals and, in turn, health professionals can disregard the priorities of patients as they make decisions about what they consider to be best for the patient. Even here, though, an appreciation of control and how it works can help people understand the dynamics of difficult situations. Grasping that perspectives differ, and how important those differences can be, could be some of the most important lessons for entering a new control paradigm of practice.

Patient-Perspective Care: A New Paradigm of Healthcare Based on Control

Perspective is so important that it warrants realigning our prevailing model of patient-centred care (Carey, 2017). What needs to be prioritised is the perspective, not the position, of the patient (Carey, 2017). Position is simply geography. For the provision of effective, efficient, and equitable health services, positioning is trivially important while perspective is critical.

The importance of perspective to effective health service delivery was starkly illustrated by a powerfully elegant study conducted almost four decades ago. Jachuck, Brierley, Jachuck, and Willcox (1982) sought to understand the impact of hypotensive drugs on a patient's quality of life. They recruited 75 consecutive patients from one group practice who all had controlled hypertension (Jachuck et al., 1982). In the study, the patients, their General Practitioners (GPs), and a close companion of each patient were asked to indicate if the hypotensive medication had improved, worsened, or had no impact on the patient's quality of life. The results were stunning (see Table 8.1). According to the GPs, all 75 patients had an improved quality of life (Jachuck et al., 1982). The close companions, however, thought that 74 patients had a *worse* quality of life, and only one patient had an improved quality of life. The perspectives of the patients were in between both these views. The opinions of 36 patients were that their quality of life had improved, 7 patients felt that their quality of life had worsened, and 32 indicated that there had been no change (Jachuck et al., 1982).

Table 8.1 Differences in perspective on patient's quality of life from Jachuck et al. (1982) and the percentage of incorrect very next treatment decisions based on that perspective

Perceived Impact on Patients' Quality of Life	**Perspective**		
	Patient	**GP**	**Close Companion**
Improved	36	75	1
Worsened	7	0	74
Unchanged	32	0	0
Next Treatment Decision Incorrect (%)	**0**	**52**	**89**

The implications of these differences in perspective are profound. Assuming that quality of life is the outcome we are most interested in, if the next treatment decision for each of these patients was based on the perspective of the GP rather than the patient, the treatment decision would be incorrect in 52% of the cases (39 patients out of 75 who didn't think their quality of life had improved). On the other hand, if the very next treatment decision was based on the close companions' opinion rather than the patients', then the treatment decision would be incorrect in 89% of the cases (67 patients out of 75 who didn't think their quality of life had deteriorated). Treatment decisions made from the perspective of patients, however, would be correct 100% of the time (see Table 8.1).

The perspective of the patient is central to eliminating health inequities by ensuring that the treatments that health professionals provide are appropriate, relevant, and desired. Prioritising the patient's perspective, however, can have important repercussions for health service delivery. In the sections below, we provide a sketch of some of the practical implications of considering people as controllers. Many of these ideas are discussed in more detail elsewhere (Carey, 2017). We should preface the offerings presented below by explaining that we are describing the general situation here where one person is voluntarily accessing a health service. Situations such as when a person has treatment mandated or is deemed to be unable to make their own decisions have important nuances that are beyond the scope of this book to explore. The general principles of what we discuss are still pertinent but the way they are applied may take some finessing.

The Golden Rule. The Golden Rule is the well-known ethos of reciprocity that is familiar in most religions and philosophies globally. Its current form is "do unto others as you would have done unto you" or "treat other people the way you want to be treated". From a "life is control" perspective, this sentiment is exactly back-to-front. A people-as-controllers Golden Rule would be "Do unto others as they would have done unto themselves" or "treat other people the way they want to be treated". We can't assume other people have the same tastes as our own.

Care. The word "care" is used indiscriminately throughout the field of health. In a control world, it would be understood that services can only legitimately be described as "care" if they are experienced as caring by the service recipients. Perhaps "care" would be more aptly used in the world of control to suggest that health professionals should take care to ensure that what they are offering as help is experienced as helpful by the helpee.

Empathy. Empathy is often touted as a highly-prized attribute in helping circles. From a people-as-controllers point of view, however, it is understood that we can never know what others are feeling. Acceptance of our own ignorance with regard to other people's emotional states can actually become an advantage when we adopt an attitude of "considered curiosity" (Carey, 2017) and tirelessly strive to find out more about another person's attitude or approach to a given situation, rather than making assumptions about them and their predicament. Regardless of how diligently we apply ourselves, we will never walk a mile, or any distance, in another person's footwear. That is not to say that we are not interested in how comfortable the person is finding their footwear or how they are experiencing the journey they are making. It is, however, only ever *their* footwear and *their* journey to experience.

Objectivity. Health professionals who understand the phenomenon of control accept that everyone has their own world view, and no-one has a privileged position where they can "objectively" consider another person's difficult situation to offer sage advice. Any time advice is given, or a particular opinion is expressed, it is granted that the opinion comes from a particular vantage point. Rather than "objectivity", the most we can strive for is impartiality or even inter-subjectivity (Velmans, 2009) when it comes to decision-making and other judgements.

Self-determination. Although the importance of self-determination is widely recognised, it is often portrayed as an important human right. From a control standpoint, however, self-determination is much more fundamental than a basic human right. The same points that we made in Chapter 4 with regard to health being a basic human right are relevant here. Self-determination is a property of the way we are designed. Digestion and thermoregulation are not considered basic human rights. Neuroplasticity is not considered a basic human right and nor is cell regeneration. It would be odd to declare that kidneys have the right to regulate electrolytes in the blood or a motor neuron has the right to transmit signals to muscle fibres across the neuromuscular junction (Carey, 2017).

First-person perspective. Health professionals who understand themselves and other people as controllers, prioritise a first-person, rather than a third-person, perspective in their work. The first-person perspective coalesces other elements we have mentioned here such as inter-subjectivity and empathy. The first-person perspective demands that the preferences, views, and opinions of the person accessing a service are the benchmarks by which decisions are made.

Standards of health. The standard approach in current healthcare is to focus, generally, on deviations from biological norms (Carey, 2017). Unfortunately, within this framework, overdiagnosis, overmedicalisation, and inappropriate care have become common (Saini et al., 2017). From a control perspective, the health professional's knowledge and understanding of ideal functioning is invaluable, however, to address health inequity, this expertise needs to be combined with the priorities of the patient to provide services that are meaningful and beneficial.

Health services. To deliver services equitably, it is critical that some groups are not being over-serviced while others are under-serviced. Focussing on the expressed needs of people seeking services with an emphasis on making services available and accessible, rather than prescribing services to them, would be the standard in a control-informed approach. A service, therefore, would be considered to be something that legitimately serves the person accessing it to help them live the life they are seeking to create.

Opportunities. It is not uncommon for health professionals to identify for patients the opportunities available to these patients in terms of potential additional assistance. The health professional might, for example, point out support groups a patient could attend or recommend specific activities they might engage in such as meditation, physical exercise, keeping a journal, or practising mindfulness. From a life is control perspective, however, anything identified as a potential opportunity would be considered an opportunity only if it helps someone better control the things that are important to them. Thus, the onus rests with the health professional to constantly strive to understand, from the perspective of the person with whom they are working, the things that are important to control for that person.

Engagement. Engagement is regularly discussed in terms of the way in which patients access and use particular services. From a control perspective, it would be assumed that everyone is always engaged in something. If patients are not "engaged" in services in the way the health professional might consider is optimal, the health professional could speculate as to what the patient *is* engaged in that is affecting, or perhaps competing with, their use of health services.

Drop-outs. Currently, people who terminate their use of services before a health professional thinks they should are typically categorised as drop-outs. In the world of control where guarding and sustaining goal states are the order of the day, the idea of dropping-out would be a misnomer. Instead, when people seem to change what it is they are pursuing at any point in time, it would be accepted that, for some reason, a different area of their experiential world has developed a bigger gap between what they want and what they're getting in that patch of their life. Rather than labelling people as drop-outs, therefore, and perhaps considering remedial action to pursue, efforts would be made to explore whether there are other aspects of the person's life that need support at this time.

Treatment effectiveness. Typically, health professionals discuss the effectiveness or otherwise of various treatments. Research programmes in fact, such as randomised controlled trials, explicitly ascribe the locus of effectiveness with the treatment or intervention and they seek to establish whether one treatment is more effective than another. Particularly with psychological and social treatments, however, it is a mistake to attribute responsibility for the production of effective outcomes with the treatment. In the bold new world of control, treatments and interventions would be understood to be resources which service providers and service recipients use to co-create desired outcomes (Carey, Fauth, & Tremblay, 2019).

Trauma. Trauma is a serious experience for some people. To be as helpful as possible to people who are traumatised, it is important to be clear about the nature of their trauma. From a control perspective, it is the inability to reconcile some aspect of highly distressing, frightening, and sometimes life-threatening, situations and events that results in what are often identified as symptoms of trauma (Carey, Mansell, Tai, & Turkington, 2014). Irreconcilable states of mind are most commonly indicative of internal conflict. As a starting point, therefore, the only assumption that might be made about someone who is taking longer to recover than they would like from a horrendously awful experience, might be that they are trapped within a conflict in their mind. A person might want, for example, to get rid of intrusive images of a past abuser so they can move on with their life while simultaneously wanting to remember the abuser so that they can erase the guilt and shame they feel. So the focus of any support or assistance would be the resolution of the conflict.

Adverse events. There is a long-established relationship between adverse events, particularly when these events occur in childhood, and the ability to live meaningful and satisfying lives as adults. Once again, adoption of a control outlook would permit a reconsideration of the attitudes of causality that are inherent in current depictions of the role of adverse events. The astute and control-minded health professional will, rather than assuming, seek to understand the nature and experience of the adversity from the perspective of the person describing the event.

It Doesn't Have to Be Difficult: Patient-Led Appointment Scheduling

A clear example of the creation, and then removal, of a situation that was inequitable in terms of access to timely treatment arose when Tim (first author) worked in the Scottish National Health Service. Through a sustained programme of research over a five-year period, Tim and his colleagues reduced the waiting time for access to receive psychological support from 15-months to less than one month by changing only the way in which appointments were scheduled. When patients, rather than clinicians, controlled the appointment scheduling there was a marked reduction in missed and cancelled appointments with the consequence being more patients were seen more of the time (Carey, 2017).

We were recently part of a team of researchers who evaluated the use of patient-led scheduling for people using specialist early intervention in psychosis services in northern England (Griffiths, Mansell, Carey, et al., 2019; Griffiths, Mansell, Edge, et al., 2019). Existing treatment guidelines recommend that people reporting psychosis should be offered 16 sessions of cognitive behavioural therapy (CBT) over a period of six months (National Institute for Health and Care Excellence (NICE), 2014). People reported appreciating the control the patient-led innovation allowed them in accessing therapy (Griffiths, Mansell, Edge, et al., 2019, p. 7), as this participant described:

> *And, I think what was nice about this was, it was very open. You had lots of, you had all these months and you could come and go as you pleased, and that flexibility was really good.*

In our view, no plausible scientific reasons have been proposed to support the recommendation that people reporting psychosis should be offered 16 sessions of CBT as opposed to any other number of sessions. Inflexible stipulations that people attend a set number of sessions fail to account for the natural variation that exists between people in terms of the duration and frequency of support they require.

In addition to addressing issues such as the appropriate frequency and duration of treatment programs, another advantage of the patient-led approach is that clinicians are free to spend less time "encouraging" people to use their services. In one study that explored experiences of the use of "assertive engagement" among healthcare professionals working in assertive outreach services (George, Manuel, Gandy-Guedes, McCray, & Negatu, 2016), one participant reported (p. 3):

> *With a lot of our clients, initially, they don't want any kind of contact with us whatsoever, and we come out regardless of how many times they slam the door in our face. We do it consistently.*

From a PCT perspective, the scenario being described in this quote is a clear example of an interpersonal conflict between a health professional and a client. Both have conflicting reference values for the state of the same variable—namely, the level of contact between each other. Efforts by one party to bring their experiences in line with their reference value have the effect of pushing the other person's experiences further away from that person's desired reference value. The more the health professional attempts to establish contact with the patient, the more dissonance this creates for the patient. The more the patient strives to alleviate their dissonance, the more the health professional's efforts will be thwarted. Leaving aside for a moment the ethics of disregarding an individual's preferences to accept or decline healthcare which have been raised as a concern (Claassen & Priebe, 2007), there are resource implications for adopting assertive approaches to engagement that are pertinent to the issue of health inequity.

How a health service or programme chooses to deploy the resources available is likely to have an effect on outcomes. The Detroit musician, Kenny Dixon Jr., makes an interesting point (Red Bull Music Academy, 2015) when he describes working creatively in the context of finite resources:

> *It ain't what you got; it's what you do with what you have, you understand?*

While we may quibble over some aspects of the sentiment expressed here, we share the view that the ways we choose to expend available resources in pursuit of a particular goal is critical in determining outcomes. This is true whether the endeavour in question relates to producing a piece of music, as in Dixon Jr's. case, or improving health outcomes. If clinicians are spending a large proportion of their time focussed on "encouraging" individuals to access or maintain contact with their service, this is necessarily time taken away from the delivery of healthcare interventions to people who are seeking to access these programs of their own volition. Keeping in mind that healthcare providers are controllers, which individual patients they decide to pursue in offering services will be influenced by the healthcare provider's own internal goals, thus potentially leading to further inequities in access to healthcare.

The issue of what constitutes "access" to healthcare is not straightforward, and a multitude of often contradictory definitions of the concept have been proposed (Oliver & Mossialos, 2004). One dimension of the concept of access, according to Gulliford et al. (2002), relates to organisational barriers which can limit access to healthcare resources. We would agree with Gulliford et al.'s (2002, p. 187) view that many barriers to access arise from a failure to use available healthcare resources efficiently and in ways that are attuned to the needs of patients:

> *Long waiting lists and waiting times may sometimes be indicative of organisational barriers to access which may result from inefficient use of existing capacity or a failure to design services around the needs of patients.*

Indeed, not only the way we conceptualise "access", but even the way we define something as a "resource", hinges on the perspective of the person for whom the "resource" is apparently relevant. With psychological treatments, for example, it is important to understand that psychologists' codes of ethics insist that people to whom services are being offered have the right to decline those services, or to withdraw from them if they have initially engaged in them (e.g. Australian Psychological Society, 2007). Meadows and Burgess (2009) investigated the "perceived need" for psychological treatments of people participating in the 2007 Australian survey of mental health and well-being. They reported that, although 20% of the sample responded in such a way that they indicated they would meet criteria for a mental health disorder within a 12-month period, only 2% of the sample indicated that they met the criteria for a mental health disorder, had a perceived need for treatment, and were not accessing services. Crucially (from our point of view), 11% of the people responding to the survey indicated that they met the criteria for a mental health disorder, were not accessing services, and *had no perceived need for treatment*. Carey and Damarell (2018, p. 10) argue that the way in which these statistics are understood and responded to in terms of resource allocation such as service provision is very closely connected to the particular framework or model to which a decision-maker or service provider subscribes:

> *Whether or not decisions are made to allocate resources to the 20% of people who meet the diagnostic criteria for a mental health disorder or to the 2% of people who meet criteria, have a perceived need for treatment, and are not accessing services, may have to do with how closely aligned decision makers are to the biomedical model. Similarly, how one responds to the 11% of people who have no perceived need for treatment but meet criteria for a mental health disorder may also depend on the particular model to which one subscribes. Health professionals who understand people to be autonomous, self-regulating agents may be comfortable with a person's right to determine how they address the difficulties they experience. Health professionals with other beliefs, however, may address the problem differently and may, for example, direct resources to engaging these people in treatment.*

We would argue that, if someone does not have a perceived need for a service or program, then it would be a mistake to describe that service or program as a resource for that person at that time.

Acknowledging People as Controllers in Our Health Policies and Models

Perhaps one of the most urgent areas for review and reformation is with policy and other documents that guide the structure of services. Policy documents need to be developed based on a sparkling and insightful appreciation of people as controllers. When an understanding of the phenomenon of control is baked into the creation of policy, the implementation of that policy is more likely to address inequities that have historically perpetuated poorer health among certain members of society. A failure to appreciate people's controlling natures can, inadvertently, lead to policies and guidelines that promote, rather than prevent, inequity.

Policies Within Health That Promote Inequity

NICE guidelines could, in many ways, be considered to provide directions that increase opportunities for inequity. NICE recommendations for the psychological treatments to be offered to people experiencing moderate depression, for example, are provided in Table 8.2 (NICE, 2009). These instructions are completely at odds with the evidence regarding patient attendance for treatment. It is well-established that most patients attend a small number of sessions and a small number of patients seek a larger number of sessions (Carey & Spratt, 2009). There is, in fact, a long-standing discrepancy between the number of sessions treatments are designed to be by clinicians and researchers, and the number of sessions that patients actually attend (Carey, 2011; Carey & Spratt, 2009).

Protocols such as the NICE Guidelines, therefore, could be contributing to lengthy waiting times as well as creating unrealistic pressure for services and health professionals (Carey, Huddy, & Griffiths, 2019). To help address inequity, through a more equitable distribution of resources, our unconditional suggestion is that these guidelines should be revised in terms of the patient-led model of service provision described above.

Table 8.2 Recommendations from the National Institute for Health and Care Excellence (NICE, 2009) regarding psychological treatment for depression

Treatment	Format	Sessions	Duration
Cognitive behavioural therapy (CBT)	Group	10 to 12	12 to 16 weeks
Cognitive behavioural therapy (CBT)	Individual	16 to 20	3 to 4 months
Interpersonal therapy	Individual	16 to 20	3 to 4 months
Behavioural activation	Individual	16 to 20	3 to 4 months
Behavioural couples therapy	Couples	15 to 20	5 to 6 months
Counselling	Individual	6 to 10	8 to 12 weeks
Psychodynamic psychotherapy	Individual	16 to 20	4 to 6 months

There's Nothing Public About Health

Since people are controllers, the experience of health, in all its varieties, will be uniquely individual. Even if the functioning of a particular organ or body part can be established with complete certainty, perhaps the level of functioning justifies a diagnosis of Type I diabetes, for example, that conviction will still reveal little about the *experience* of the condition for each individual.

It is imperative that, in our policies and guidelines, we become much better at advocating for the organisation of resources, circumstances, and conditions, so individuals can arrange their affairs in the manner that suits them. While individuals may gather together in large and small groups, it is never the group that experiences a health problem. We need to get much better at distinguishing between the mass and the units that make up the mass. This well-circulated story poignantly captures the sentiment we are championing without reservation here:

> *One day a man was walking along the beach when he noticed a boy picking something up and gently throwing it into the ocean. Approaching the boy, he asked,*
>
> *"What are you doing?"*
>
> *The youth replied,*
>
> *"Throwing starfish back into the ocean. The surf is up and the tide is going out. If I don't throw them back, they'll die."*
>
> *"Son,"*
>
> *the man said,*
>
> *"don't you realize there are miles and miles of beach and hundreds of starfish? You can't make a difference!"*
>
> *After listening politely, the boy bent down, picked up another starfish, and threw it back into the surf. Then, smiling at the man, he said...*
>
> *"I made a difference for that one."*[1]

Our attention should focus much more on "making a difference for that one". Health is an individual affair. Or, to be more precise, accurate, and consistent with PCT, we need to concentrate on organising events and affairs so that individuals have the necessary degrees of freedom to make whatever differences they want to experience when and as they need to make them.

[1] http://www.ataturksociety.org/the-starfish-story-original-story-by-loren-eisley/.

Perhaps the most dangerous idea in society is the belief by one person, that they know what is best for another. Being savy to our controlling natures necessitates registering that we never know what is best for another person and we need to stop pretending that we do. Any pronouncement of a "best" course of action must always be brought before the goals and intended outcomes for whom this course is being bestowed. Is option A better for patient X than option B. The spirit of "It depends" to which we have previously referred is profound in its simplicity and accuracy. The relevance of any advisement is always contingent upon the way a person wants things to be.

We have now explored both the research and practice implications of diverting our gaze from inequity to control. We have almost come to the end of the tale of our journey to the centre of the health inequity field and back again. In the final chapter, we highlight and summarise some of our main points in a general sense to convey an unequivocal message for society. To be sure, we are just as much in the dark about the ultimate landscape as we expect you might be. We have some reasoned assumptions, and one or two clear ideas of the direction to take. The genuinely exciting aspect of the manifesto we are peddling, however, is that the destination is yet to be created. The key is control, and we all can have the key. Having the key, however, is meaningless unless we turn it. The adventures and discoveries of a world of control are now within our reach, but we must do the reaching.

References

Australian Psychological Society. (2007). *Code of ethics*. Melbourne: Australian Psychological Society.

Burns, H. (2014). What causes health? *Journal of the Royal College of Physicians of Edinburgh, 44*, 103–105.

Carey, T. A. (2011). As you like it: Adopting a patient-led approach to the issue of treatment length. *Journal of Public Mental Health, 10*(1), 6–16.

Carey, T. A. (2016). Health is control. *Annals of Behavioural Science, 2*(13), 1–3. Accessed 12 September 2020. https://behaviouralscience.imedpub.com/health-is-control.php?aid=8637.

Carey, T. A. (2017). *Patient-perspective care: A new paradigm for health systems and services*. London: Routledge.

Carey, T. A., & Damarell, R. A. (2018). A systematic review investigating the comparative effectiveness and efficiency of a multi clinician stepped care workforce Vs. a single clinician stepped care workforce for delivering psychological treatments. *Annals of Behavioural Science, 4*(2), 1–6. https://doi.org/10.21767/2471-7975.100034.

Carey, T. A., Fauth, J. M., & Tremblay, G. T. (2019). Rethinking evaluation for improved health outcomes: Implications for remote Australia. *American Journal of Evaluation,* 1–21. https://doi.org/10.1177/1098214018824040.

Carey, T. A., Huddy, V., & Griffiths, R. (2019). To mix or not to mix? A meta-method approach to rethinking evaluation practices for improved effectiveness and efficiency of psychological therapies illustrated with the application of perceptual control theory. *Frontiers in Psychology, 10,* 1445.

Carey, T. A., Mansell, W., Tai, S. J., & Turkington, D. (2014). Conflicted control systems: The neural architecture of trauma. *Lancet Psychiatry, 1,* 316–318.

Carey, T. A., & Spratt, M. B. (2009). When is enough enough? Structuring the organisation of treatment to maximise patient choice and control. *The Cognitive Behaviour Therapist, 2,* 211–226.

Claassen, D., & Priebe, S. (2007). Ethical aspects of assertive outreach. *Psychiatry, 6*(2), 45–48. https://doi.org/10.1016/j.mppsy.2006.11.007.

George, M., Manuel, J. I., Gandy-Guedes, M. E., McCray, S., & Negatu, D. (2016). "Sometimes what they think is helpful is not really helpful": Understanding engagement in the program of assertive community treatment (PACT). *Community Mental Health Journal, 52*(8), 882–890. https://doi.org/10.1007/s10597-015-9934-9.

Griffiths, R., Mansell, W., Carey, T. A., Edge, D., Emsley, R., & Tai, S. J. (2019). Method of levels therapy for first-episode psychosis: The feasibility randomized controlled Next Level trial. *Journal of Clinical Psychology, 75*(10), 1756–1769. https://doi.org/10.1002/jclp.22820.

Griffiths, R., Mansell, W., Edge, D., Carey, T. A., Peel, H., & Tai, S. J. (2019). 'It was me answering my own questions': Experiences of method of levels therapy amongst people with first-episode psychosis. *International Journal of Mental Health Nursing, 28*(3), 1–14. https://doi.org/10.1111/inm.12576.

Gulliford, M., Figueroa-Munoz, J., Morgan, M., Hughes, D., Gibson, B., Beech, R., & Hudson, M. (2002). What does "access to health care" mean? *Journal of Health Services Research and Policy, 7*(3), 186–188. https://doi.org/10.1258/135581902760082517.

Jachuck, S. J., Brierley, H., Jachuck, S., & Willcox, P. M. (1982). The effect of hypotensive drugs on the quality of life. *Journal of the Royal College of General Practitioners, 32,* 103–105.

Marken, R. S. (1988). The nature of behavior: Control as fact and theory. *Behavioral Science, 33*(3), 196–206. https://doi.org/10.1002/bs.3830330304.

Marken, R. S., & Carey, T. A. (2015). *Controlling people: The paradoxical nature of being human.* Brisbane: Australian Academic Press.

Meadows, G. N., & Burgess, P. M. (2009). Perceived need for mental health care: Findings from the 2007 Australian survey of mental health and wellbeing. *Australian and New Zealand Journal of Psychiatry, 43,* 624–634.

NICE. (2009). *Depression in adults: Recognition and management. Clinical guideline [CG90].* Accessed 12 September 2020. https://www.nice.org.uk/guidance/cg90/ifp/chapter/Treatments-for-mild-to-moderate-depression.

NICE. (2014). *Psychosis and schizophrenia in adults: Prevention and management. Clinical guidelines [CG178].* Accessed 6 March 2021. https://www.nice.org.uk/guidance/cg178/chapter/recommendations#how-to-deliver-psychological-interventions.

Oliver, A., & Mossialos, E. (2004). Equity of access to health care: Outlining the foundations for action. *Journal of Epidemiology and Community Health, 58*(8), 655–658. https://doi.org/10.1136/jech.2003.017731.

Red Bull Music Academy. (2015, May 7). *Moodymann talks detroit and being independent* [Video File]. Accessed 12 September 2020. https://www.youtube.com/watch?v=6MURWcoKrWI&feature=youtu.be.

Saini, V., Garcia-Armesto, S., Klemperer, D., Paris, V., Elshaug, A. G., Brownlee, S., … Fisher, E. S. (2017). *Drivers of poor medical care.* Lancet, Published online 8 January. http://dx.doi.org/10.1016/S0140-6736(16)30947-3.

Velmans, M. (2009). *Understanding consciousness* (2nd ed.). London: Routledge.

CHAPTER 9

Well That's That Then. We're All Controllers All Controlling Together. So What?

The childhood of the human race is far from over. We have a long way to go before most people will understand that what they do for others is just as important to their wellbeing as what they do for themselves. William T. Powers

So here we are. We began this book by explaining that, for us, some of the claims being made in the health inequity literature didn't add up. This book has been somewhat of a chronicling of our efforts to make sense of the field in the context of a particular theory of living of which we have been students for a number of decades.

Our purpose in writing this work was straightforward and twofold. First, we wanted to highlight what we saw as shortcomings, limitations, and contradictions in the health inequity domain. Second, we wanted to offer Perceptual Control Theory (PCT; Powers, 1973, 2005) as a possible framework for improving the cohesiveness, clarity, and progress of the discipline.

We wanted to highlight problems that we saw in how health inequity is currently understood and investigated. We think the current research and theory building habits are limitations that are severely restricting the extent to which the field is advancing. We unreservedly believe that PCT has something to offer. From our perspective, PCT holds the promise of opening a door to a world that is less inequitable by orders of magnitude than the current inequity at our global address.

T. A. Carey et al., *Deconstructing Health Inequity*,
https://doi.org/10.1007/978-3-030-68053-4_9

While we are in no doubt of the potential benefit that a PCT approach suggests, we are also acutely aware that PCT's promise is a new direction and a new journey for researchers, practitioners, and policy- and other decision-makers. PCT is not a prescriptive theory that defines a clear solution. Rather, it provides a genuinely novel point of view from which to consider the questions we regard as important as well as the way we go about answering them.

We fully acknowledge that we are relative newcomers to the health inequity domain. For that reason, we have endeavoured throughout the book to concentrate our efforts on the area we know best—PCT. We believe our most useful contribution is to outline the way in which a control perspective can be applied to health inequity. In the final analysis, we are probably not the best judges of this assumption.

No doubt, throughout this book, various topics have been highlighted that could have been explored in far greater detail. In different places, and to differing degrees, our discussions have been wide-ranging and included matters such as economics, research methods, modelling, and policy development. While we have some interest in each of these, and other areas, they are not fields in which we feel we have specialist, advanced knowledge and expertise. We hope we have offered sufficient information and resources from a PCT perspective so that others have the beginnings of what they need to pursue this line of enquiry if they wish to.

This book, therefore, is both an invitation and a challenge. In the paragraphs below, we will recap on the main points of each chapter by explaining our choice of each opening chapter quote. We will conclude by returning to the quote that began this chapter and leave you with our views on the ultimate implications for building a world where social living, and all that it entails, is understood as control.

The True Measure of Any Society Can Be Found in How It Treats Its Most Vulnerable Members

Gandhi's wisdom with which we chose to open the first chapter could be considered to exemplify the inequity ethos. The potency of his standard is just as relevant today. On the Partners in Health website, for example, the quote "The idea that some lives matter less is the root of all that is wrong with the world"[1] is attributed to the medical anthropologist Professor Paul Farmer. Farmer is a co-founder of Partners in Health and Chair of the Department of Global Health and Social Medicine at Harvard University Medical School. The original source of the quote appears to be Kidder's (2011) biography of Farmer *Mountains Beyond Mountains*. The complete prose is:

> *And I can imagine Farmer saying he doesn't care if no one else is willing to follow their example. He's still going to make these hikes, he'd insist, because if you say that seven hours is too long to walk for two families of patients, you're saying that their lives matter less than some others', and the idea that some lives matter less is the root of all that's wrong with the world.* (p. 294)

While we completely concur with the message being conveyed in this quote, we wonder whether a slight rewording might be even more accurate:

> *The idea that some lives matter more is the root of all that is wrong with the world.*

Although this might seem like an inconsequential change, it is actually the advantaging of some, through government initiatives such as inequitable taxation and other policies, that results in inequity. Lives mattering less appears to arise as a byproduct of the deeds of politicians, policy- and other decision-makers, which seem to unequivocally demonstrate that they believe that some lives matter more. Stiglitz and Bilmes (2012), for example, suggest that when one group holds an imbalance of power, the group can develop and introduce policies that favour it in the short term. In the United States (US) today, there is a widening gap between the wealthiest 1% and everyone else. Stiglitz (2011) insists that inequity exists, because the top 1% want it to. Gandhi might suggest that such a society is privileging its wealthy at the expense of its most vulnerable.

You might recognise by now that the creation and maintenance of inequity is a control process. The top 1% have an extravagant abundance of resources that enable them to arrange economic and social conditions in the ways that suit them best. Currently in the US, most politicians are members of the top 1% club as are many policymakers

[1] www.pih.org.

concerned with economic and trade policy (Stiglitz, 2011). While the argument could be advanced that the top 1 percenters don't actually set out to *directly* disadvantage the rest, it is their short-sighted fixation with securing and expanding their own fabulous fortunes from which the disadvantage arises. Inequity can be understood as a side effect of the myopically focussed controlling of a tiny band of mightily powerful individuals.

It is a small group of powerful people who seem irrefutably to be of the opinion that their lives matter more which is the root of our current inequity problems. Self-interest, per se, is not the problem. We will have more to say about self-interest below. It might be beneficial to foreshadow the later discussion, however, with the suggestion that PCT explains *all* interest as, ultimately, self-interest. The only reason anyone does anything at all is to either maintain some state of their experiential world as it is or to rectify an aspect that has suffered a blip. Even the most benevolent or selfless seeming acts are driven by the irrepressible urge to maintain an individual's ticker-tape report of reality in line with their internal standards. This is the case whether the apparently philanthropic act involves huge charitable donations or diving headfirst into a river to rescue a struggling swimmer. So, self-interest is not the problem. Where that self-interest is focussed, however, can either attenuate or exacerbate problems such as inequity depending on the resources one is able to mobilise.

We spent the first chapter outlining some of the most prominent themes in the health inequity literature. We thought it was important to begin by explaining that despite the recency of our arrival to the health inequity arena, themes of social justice and equity have been important to us for a long time. From our initial reading of the health inequity literature, we were perplexed by some of the statements being made and we wanted to figure out why inequity should *necessarily* be a problem as well as why it might be so difficult to resolve.

We outlined some of the major discrepancies in the literature and we introduced an idea that became somewhat of a theme throughout the book. The idea was that a change in perspective might be very useful for the inequity field to establish greater cohesion and clarity. This book, in fact, could be described as the detailed outlining of a suggested new direction for health inequity research, policy, and practice.

Scientists Have Learned to Respect Nothing but Evidence, and to Believe that Their Highest Duty Lies in Submitting to It However It May Jar Against Their Inclinations

We chose the quote by Thomas Huxley for the second chapter because it seemed to be especially relevant in terms of depicting the way in which knowledge was being amassed in the health inequity field and what might possibly help to move the field forward. In important areas such as theory development, methodological considerations, and the clarity of key concepts, there seemed to be more of a mindset of advancing particular ideologies and beliefs rather than using rigorous approaches in the conduct of empirical work. Personally, we were sympathetic with many of the views being proposed. At the same time, however, we thought greater attention to a scientific attitude (McIntyre, 2019) with this body of work might help to progress the field. McIntyre (2019) is unequivocal in this regard. He asserts that "To do science we must be willing to embrace a mindset that tells us that our prior beliefs, ideologies, and wishes do not matter in deciding what can pass the test of comparison with the evidence" (p. 17).

In this chapter, specific attention was devoted to some selected findings to highlight particular claims being made. From the research we consulted, it seemed to us that the way in which some conclusions were described didn't always seem to closely map onto the actual results that had been obtained. For us, this was an important point to clarify in order to have some appreciation of what the state of knowledge actually was in this area.

Facts Are Stubborn Things, and Whatever May Be Our Wishes, Our Inclinations, or the Dictums of Our Passions, They Cannot Alter the State of Facts and Evidence

Since we are claiming that control is a fact of nature, we considered this quote by John Adams was particularly apt for the third chapter. The PCT attitude is that control is the process of living. Anyone who is alive, therefore, is controlling. People are still controlling even if they don't know they are. Activities such as selecting theories and building programs of research are control processes whether or not the theories and research are about control or something else entirely.

Appreciating how control works according to the process of negative feedback delivers some surprises for the way in which we understand behaviour. In this chapter, we discussed the implications of a PCT approach for areas such as the way in which we conceptualise, describe, and discuss mechanisms as well as our understanding of causality. By the time we had wound our way to the end of this chapter, we felt comfortably justified in concluding that inequity per se was not the problem. The problem, always, is compromised control. It is compromised control, therefore, that needs to be addressed and rectified. Targetting inequity will not necessarily improve control, however, correcting whatever control problems exist will, simultaneously, remove any associated inequity issues.

The Habit of an Opinion Often Leads to the Complete Conviction of Its Truth, It Hides the Weaker Parts of It, and Makes Us Incapable of Accepting the Proofs Against It

The quote by Jons Jacob Berzelius for this chapter is one of many examples we frequently encounter in which people quite accurately depict control processes while seeming to be unaware that they are doing this. In many ways, PCT predicts its own rejection! PCT principles and assumptions are orthogonal to many widely accepted beliefs and attitudes in the behavioural sciences. When ideas are encountered for the first time which clash with existing notions of the way things are, the habit of a controlling entity is to do whatever needs to be done to remove those jarring effects.

Marks (2000), whose work we mentioned in Chapter Three writes lucidly and unambiguously that "Our beliefs are not automatically updated by the best available evidence. They often have an active life of their own and fight tenaciously for their own survival" (p. 259). Richard Wiseman is another authority who captures the sentiment of underlying control processes maintaining a homeostatic equilibrium in our cognitive milieu. According to Wiseman "Our beliefs do not sit passively in our brains waiting to be confirmed or contradicted by incoming information. Instead, they play a key role in shaping how we see the world".[2]

We were very aware throughout the writing of this book that many of our suggestions would invite opposition and counteracting by some readers. We often found ourselves, therefore, in a dilemma between wanting to clearly describe the potential that we think PCT has to offer but also wanting to connect with prevailing standards and norms. Babies and bathwater were constantly on our minds during our deliberations and musings. We strived to adopt an attitude of raising possibilities and identifying areas that could be candidates to be considered for reform. The way in which we currently define health is one of those areas and, in this chapter, we suggest that there could be merit in defining health as control.

Truth Does not Change Because It Is, or Is not Believed by a Majority of the People

To enable people to have an expanded appreciation of some of the implications of what embracing the idea of living as control might encompass, we thought it would be helpful to focus on a small number of key areas. Some of the most basic assumptions with regard to matters such as causality would be radically overhauled, and other areas such as researchers' goals and decision-making would have a much greater focus and be more carefully scrutinised in a world where control was understood to be the only show in town. Science, however, is not a consensus enterprise or a popularity contest. Ideas should be judged, and either retained or rejected based on merit, not according to how many people subscribe to them as Giordano Bruno's quote indicates. Science also evolves and improves over time (Zimring, 2019). It is our conviction that the long-term benefits of drastically modifying the concepts we identified and their current positions of dominance would more than justify the initial discomfort of reorganising existing belief structures.

This conviction, however, is something we recognise as ours and ours alone. The extent to which other people might be similarly impressed with control ideas is something of which we are ignorant. Yet we understand everybody to be controllers. We thought it would be helpful, therefore, to

[2] https://quotes.pub/q/our-beliefs-do-not-sit-passively-in-our-brains-waiting-to-be-542033.

spend some time raising an awareness of some of what being a controlling researcher entails. A raised awareness provides an opportunity for people to do what they want to do even better than before if they are not satisfied with their current activity and results.

In Questions of Science, the Authority of a Thousand Is not Worth the Humble Reasoning of a Single Individual

The current way in which we conduct statistical analyses would change in a world where control was the phenomenon of interest. There would be a much clearer distinction between correlation and causation and a sophisticated and nuanced understanding of the scope and limitations of conclusions that are deemed to be statistically significant. In a world where people were recognised as controllers there would also be a move away from an almost complete reliance on aggregated data for making decisions and conclusions about the way in which people function.

We definitely do not want to leave you with the impression that models and methods don't matter. We think they matter tremendously which is why we think that all deliberations regarding the construction of models and the appropriate choice of methods for any given program of research should occur within the context of an accurate understanding of how we are designed. The spirit of Galileo Galilei's quote is that it matters to get it right. Our suggestion throughout this book is that understanding control and applying the principles of PCT are ways of pursuing "right" and getting it more right than we ever have before. It's a way of raising the bar for scientific activity in the behavioural sciences.

We Have to Live Today by What Truth We Can Get Today, and Be Ready Tomorrow to Call It Falsehood

We thought this quote by William James captured the evolving nature of science mentioned above and resonated strongly with the promise of PCT to illuminate a different and more productive path. While science undoubtedly aims at discovering empirical truths, it also comfortably accommodates uncertainty within the knowledge that whatever is considered the most accurate truth today, might be revised or overturned tomorrow based on new empirical data (McIntyre, 2019).

PCT offers an avenue for establishing contemporary truths as well as exploring what the truths of tomorrow might become. As a way of illustrating what small steps in a PCT direction might be, we took somewhat of a case study approach in this chapter. We spent time sifting through the report of one particular study. Our efforts here were not intended to demean or belittle this research in any way. Rather, we think this was an important piece of work for the today of its time. From our impressions of what a PCT tomorrow could offer, however, we spotlighted some of the areas in which a recognition of people as controllers might have taken the research in a profoundly different direction.

I Cannot Say Whether Things Will Get Better if We Change; What I Can Say Is They Must Change if They Are to Get Better

The epigraph by George C. Lichtenberg that heralded the ensuing theme of Chapter 8, also encapsulated the entire character of the book in which we do what we can to describe a different perspective as an invitation to consider an alternative approach for the opportunity to make things radically better. We recognise our focus throughout this book emphasises research and policy more than practice. Our emphasis perhaps reflects the focus of the literature we encountered and considered. There are quite important, specific, and tangible lessons, however, for health professionals and other practitioners seeking to address health inequity.

In this chapter, we provide some suggestions from our own experiences as practising health professionals with regard to the attitudinal and practical transformations that can be beneficial. In particular, shifting from a patient-centred to a patient-perspective framework (Carey, 2017) is likely to yield important dividends. There is still much work to be done, with many questions yet to be asked and answered. Nevertheless, there is a growing body of work that can provide useful suggestions and indicators for reform if practitioners and health service managers recognise that such a manoeuver is warranted.

The Childhood of the Human Race Is Far from Over. We Have a Long Way to Go Before Most People Will Understand that What They Do for Others Is Just as Important to Their Wellbeing as What They Do for Themselves

It was fitting that a quote from William T. Powers should frame the last chapter. The profoundly prophetic nature of these words, however, might not initially be grasped. The sentiment expressed in these sentences captures the dilemma of being a controlling agent in the midst of a legion of controlling agents. The fact that we are designed to control but also to resist being controlled has been described as the paradoxical nature of being human (Marken & Carey, 2015).

The idea that our own well-being is inextricably bound to the well-being of others is not just a schmaltzy decree designed to persuade people to play nicely together in our terrestrial sandpit. While the quote might seem like a suitable title for a motivational poster, perhaps accompanied by groups of people engaged in wholesome share activities, like rowing or volunteering for the cake stall at the school fair, it actually reflects something fundamental about our controlling natures. Given our assemblage according to the control system blueprint, our ability to control the things that are important to us is heavily influenced by the degrees of freedom we are afforded in the environments in which we dwell. As control systems, we want, and we push back (Carey, 2020). The less people get what they want, the more they will push back. The unpreventable pushing back will interfere with the controlling of others which will result in still more push-back. It is *necessarily* the case, therefore, that what we do for others is just as important to our well-being as what we do for ourselves.

At first glance, this idea might seem to be a restating of the widespread notion of reciprocity. There is a subtlety here, however, that makes this declaration decisively and monumentally distinct. Whereas reciprocity promotes a kind of "I'll scratch your back if you scratch mine", or even "I'll scratch your back because mine will need scratching later and I know you'll be there to call on", in Powers pronouncement, the suggestion is to do for others *regardless* of what they do for you.

The value in moving beyond the simplicity of reciprocity has been captured by others. Stiglitz (2011), for example, refers to Alexis de

Tocqueville's (1835) *Democracy in America* in which he refers to "self-interest rightly understood". PCT can contribute some scientific rigour to the "rightly understood" aspect of this phrase. As controllers, everything we do is for the purpose of making or keeping some aspect of our experiential world in the state we have specified it must be. In the final analysis, a tireless charity worker, or some other citizen identified as altruistic in the extreme, behaves the way they do to keep their worlds the way they must be. To behave in any other way would, sooner or later, generate internal conflict for them. This is the self-interest to which earlier we promised we would return.

Stiglitz (2011) may be unaware of the phenomenon of control but he is astute enough to sense the colossal gravity of these ideas. He relates them directly to inequity. Stiglitz (2011) expresses it in a way that might not be palatable for some:

> *... looking out for the other guy isn't just good for the soul—it's good for business.*

Stiglitz (2011) explains that the fate of those in the top 1% of incomes is inherently coupled to the fate of the remaining 99%. He reminds us that, throughout history, those in the stratosphere of wealth have only learned this lesson when it was too late. Will history repeat itself again? Now, with the science of PCT we have the possibility of embarking on a new adventure. We have it in our grasp to forge a different future for ourselves. Will we be brave enough to step out. On this point, Stiglitz and Bilmes (2012) are unequivocal:

> *... there comes a point when inequality spirals into economic dysfunction for the whole society, and when it does, even the rich pay a steep price.*

They go on to explain their stance in unambiguous terms:

> *So, the advice I'd give to the 1 percent today is: Harden your hearts. When invited to consider proposals to reduce inequality—by raising taxes and investing in education, public works, health care, and science—put any latent notions of altruism aside and reduce the idea to one of unadulterated self-interest. Don't embrace it because it helps other people. Just do it for yourself.* (Stiglitz & Bilmes, 2012)

Economies with the greatest inequities might be regarded as all tip and no iceberg. The tip forgets its iceberg at its peril. It might enjoy its moment in the sun but a moment may be all it has. A failure to attend to, and nurture, bases and foundational structures is never a sustainable situation.

The so What of It All

There seems little else to say at this point. Unadulterated self-interest might be something for which people are willing to sign on the dotted line. Inequity is bad because it interferes with control. Control is as essential to life as breathing. We can restrict people's breathing for a period of time, but we can't stop them gasping for breath and seeking fresh air. Currently, globally, our kind is gasping for breath and seeking fresh air.

Health inequity may well be the miner's canary which is bellowing the message that people's ability to control is being dangerously obstructed. Dangerous for the individuals and their welfare undoubtedly, but also dangerous for the longevity of our economies and communities. The difference this time in the annals of human history, however, is that we have the technology to understand our design and to begin to develop solutions that are compatible with, rather than antagonistic to, that design.

With PCT, the answers are not yet in sight. In fact, the questions have barely begun to be formed. There are just the very earliest indications of a new day emerging on the horizon of health and social living. Whether we turn towards the softening light to explore what possibilities we might create for ourselves, or stay meandering along in the comfort of the dark, is an individual decision. The repercussions of the decision, however, will be unavoidable. We cannot escape the inescapable.

Controlling is inevitable and unavoidable. To safeguard our own controlling, we must attend to the controlling of others. Inequity signals the presence of a problem, but it is not, itself, the problem to be solved. Living together as controllers is the problem to be solved. It is a problem that has been a dogged and relentless companion of our race since group living first began. We have now been gifted with the chance to gaze anew at our plight. Though this fresh perspective might initially seem blurry and disorienting, as more and more elements of social living are brought into focus through the lens of control, we might finally understand how we can most thoroughly help ourselves.

How can societies be arranged such that there are sufficient degrees of freedom for all residents to control the things that are important to themselves without preventing others from doing the same thing? An answer to that question might reveal the unlimited magnificence of all that a group of controllers can achieve.

References

Carey, T. A. (2017). *Patient-perspective care: A new paradigm for health systems and services*. London: Routledge. https://doi.org/10.4324/9781351227988.

Carey, T. A. (2020, August 14). Who cares what others want? You should! For your own sake. *Psychology Today*. Accessed 15 September 2020. https://www.psychologytoday.com/intl/blog/in-control/202008/who-cares-what-others-want.

Kidder, T. (2011). *Mountains beyond mountains: One doctor's quest to heal the world*. London: Profile Books.

Marken, R. S., & Carey, T. A. (2015). *Controlling people: The paradoxical nature of being human*. Brisbane: Australian Academic Press.

Marks, D. F. (2000). *The psychology of the psychic* (2nd ed.). Amherst, NY: Prometheus Books.

McIntyre, L. (2019). *The scientific attitude: Defending science from denial, fraud, and pseudoscience*. Cambridge, MA: Massachusetts Institute of Technology.

Powers, W. T. (1973). *Behavior: The control of perception*. Chicago: Aldine.

Powers, W. T. (2005). *Behavior: The control of perception* (2nd ed.). New Canaan, CT: Benchmark.

Stiglitz, J. (2011, March 31). Of the 1%, by the 1%, for the 1%. *Vanity Fair*. Accessed 12 September 2020. https://www.vanityfair.com/news/2011/05/top-one-percent-201105.

Stiglitz, J., & Bilmes, L. J. (2012, May 31). The 1 percent's problem. *Vanity Fair*. Accessed 12 September 2020. https://www.vanityfair.com/news/2012/05/joseph-stiglitz-the-price-on-inequality.

Zimring, J. C. (2019). *What science is and how it really works*. Cambridge, UK: Cambridge University Press.

Index

T. A. Carey et al., *Deconstructing Health Inequity*,
https://doi.org/10.1007/978-3-030-68053-4

CPSIA information can be obtained
at www.ICGtesting.com
Printed in the USA
LVHW021718030521
686345LV00003B/255

9 783030 680527